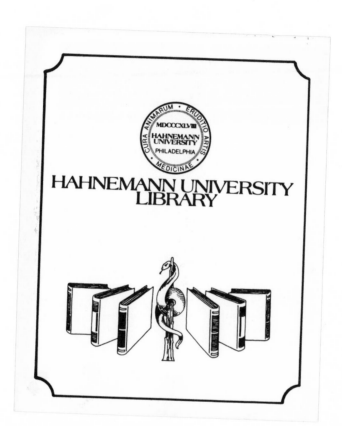

Atlas of
Amputation Surgery

Atlas of
Amputation Surgery

WALTHER H.O. BOHNE, M.D., F.A.C.S.
Hospital for Special Surgery
New York, New York

With 253 illustrations

Medical Illustrations by William Thackeray

1987
Thieme Medical Publishers, Inc., New York
Georg Thieme Verlag, Stuttgart · New York

Thieme Medical Publishers, Inc.
381 Park Avenue South
New York, New York 10016

Cover design by Nancy Widdows

ATLAS OF AMPUTATION SURGERY
Walther H.O. Bohne

Library of Congress Cataloging-in-Publication Data
Bohne, Walther H.O.
    Atlas of amputation surgery.

    Includes index.
    1. Amputation. 2. Amputation—Atlases. I. Title.
[DNLM: 1. Amputation—atlases. WE 17 B677a]
RD553.B64 1987   617′.58   87-6533

Important note: Medicine is an ever-changing science. Research and clinical experience are con-
tinually broadening our knowledge, in particular our knowledge of proper treatment and drug
therapy. Insofar as this book mentions any dosage or application, readers may rest assured that the
authors, editors, and publishers have made every effort to ensure that such references are strictly in
accordance with the state of knowledge at the time of production of the book. Nevertheless, every
user is requested to carefully examine the manufacturers' leaflets accompanying each drug to
check on his own responsibility whether the dosage schedules recommended therein or the contraindications stated by the manufacturers differ from the statements made in the present book.
Such examination is particularly important with drugs that are either rarely used or have been
newly released on the market.

Some of the product names, patents, and registered designs referred to in this book are in fact
registered trademarks or proprietary names even though specific reference to this fact is not always
made in the text. Therefore, the appearance of a name without designation as proprietary is not to
be construed as a representation by the publisher that it is in the public domain.

Printed in the United States of America.

5   4   3   2   1

TMP ISBN 0-86577-125-1
GTV ISBN 3-13-652801-1

Preface

Amputation surgery has changed rather dramatically over the last 150 years. While only a few new procedures have been added to the armamentarium of surgeons, the advances in surgery and medicine have resulted in a change in emphasis on various aspects of the procedures. Speed is no longer of the essence, and preselected levels of amputation have given way to the ideas of conserving tissue and improving strength, stability, and function of the remaining part of the limb. While most amputations were open amputations until the advent of asepsis and antisepsis, the opposite is currently true, although the open amputation has maintained its place in a number of areas. Most important, however, any amputation performed today should be undertaken not only with the plan to eradicate disease, but with a long-term plan for ultimate prosthetic fitting as well as the physical and emotional rehabilitation of the patient.

The decision to amputate should be made with reluctance and only after consultation with other physicians, which should be sought whenever possible. However, where amputation must be performed, the surgeon should have intimate knowledge of the procedure intended, its pitfalls, and its ultimate consequences for the patient. Beyond that, as in so many procedures carried out repeatedly, the surgeon will develop personal preferences and idiosyncrasies. These preferences are the mainstay of this book, although every attempt has been made to present a balanced picture. If a procedure, or variation of a procedure, has not been presented, it has been due more to the number of possible approaches for the anatomic site, rather than a reflection of their value.

This preface would not be complete without giving thanks to those who helped with the preparation of this book:

Mr. William Thackeray invested much time and effort in preparing the illustrations. And, even though I often despaired about ever receiving the final drafts, he ultimately came through.

I owe much thanks to Dr. Seidman for the chapter, "Anesthesia."

I must express special thanks to Dr. Richard McCormick, who reviewed the chapters on finger and hand amputation and gave valuable help.

Mr. Raymond Mis helped with the compilation of bibliographies for which I express my gratitude.

There are people who combine the patience of Job with the disposition of a parent of a three-year-old child. They had faith in the ultimate completion of the project and, at the same time, were able to urge on the disparing author. I was fortunate enough to find these characteristics in the three people I worked with at Thieme Medical Publishers: Brian Decker, early in the planning stages of the book, but particularly Jill Rudansky and Jim Costello throughout the completion of the book. Without their help and involvement, I should have been inclined to give up several times.

Special thanks go to Ms. Cynthia Pardue for the many times she retyped the manuscript.

Walther H.O. Bohne

Murdoch G: Amputation revisited. The Knud Jansen lecture. Department of Orthopaedic and Traumatic Surgery, University of Dundee, Scotland. Prosthetics and Orthotics Int 8:8–15, 1984.

Slocum, DB: An Atlas of Amputation. CV Mosby Co., 1949.

Foreword

This text/atlas should serve as an important resource for currently practicing surgeons. At present, we are in an era so dominated by surgical concepts of limb conservation and restoration that the surgeon is ill prepared to face the challenge of an amputation when it is indicated. A logically organized reference of this kind, therefore, should be at hand on every surgeon's book shelf.

The comprehensive nature of this text/atlas should also supply the serious student of amputations with all the current information needed for understanding the modern concepts of this traditional but changing field of surgery —from indications to long-term care.

This text/atlas is written by an experienced orthopedic surgeon who is particularly knowledgeable in the field of prosthetics. Therefore, the principles of surgical management discussed in this book are governed by postoperative considerations of stump care, prosthetic fitting, rehabilitation, and practical outcome objectives.

I strongly recommend this *Atlas of Amputation Surgery* not only to all surgeons and surgical students, but also to those in ancillary professions who are concerned with the care of amputees.

Philip D. Wilson, Jr., M.D.

Contents

Part III. Postoperative Considerations

Part One
General Considerations

CHAPTER 1
Indications for Amputation

In 1968, Burgess and Romano[1] showed in a simple graph the distribution of indications for amputation in 160 cases of lower extremity amputees who were divided into age groups. In the 1 to 12 year age group, the main reason for amputation was a congenital defect. The only other indications for amputations were post-traumatic complications. This latter indication increased in number in the 13 to 24 year age group. A close second was malignant disease, while congenital defects and infection played lesser roles. Between the ages of 25 and 50 years, infection and post-traumatic complications were the indications in the majority of cases; however, vascular disease with or without diabetes became an increasingly frequent cause for amputation. The 51 to 75 year age group constituted the largest number of amputees in this study. Of these, most were amputated for reasons of vascular disease; infection and malignant disease played a lesser role. Vascular disease remained the main reason for lower extremity amputations in patients above 75 years of age.

In two large survey studies,[2,3] the causes for amputation were grouped under the following four categories (Table 1-1):

1. *Trauma* was the cause when amputations were done because of physical or thermal injuries, and because of infections following the injury.
2. *Disease* was cited as the cause for amputation when vascular diseases or infections were present.
3. *Tumors* were considered the cause when the amputation was done for benign or malignant growths.
4. *Congenital amputations* were considered only in cases where prostheses were fitted. The type of prosthesis used also determined the level of amputation.

Table 1-1. Ratios of Males to Females in Relation to Cause of Amputation*

	Current Study	Glattly Study
Trauma	7.2 – 1.0	9.2 – 1.0
Disease	2.1 – 1.0	2.6 – 1.0
Tumor	1.3 – 1.0	1.2 – 1.0
Congenital	1.5 – 1.0	1.2 – 1.0

* Reprinted by permission from Kay and Newman.[3]

In this particular study, no differentiation between upper and lower extremities was made. Distribution by cause and sex can be seen in Figure 1-1. However, considerable disparity between the upper and lower extremity amputation did exist (Fig. 1-2).

In the developed countries, the increasing age of the population contributes to the development of diseases leading to amputations. Vascular insufficiency and diabetes mellitus have long since become the leading causes for lower extremity amputations. In the United States, no comprehensive studies are available for the last 10 years on the etiology of lower extremity amputations. An estimate is that around 80% are done for reasons of vascular insufficiency. This figure is supported by statistics from other countries. An example is a survey of the Danish Amputation Register, which shows us that the reason for 2,404 major amputations in the lower extremity performed in 1980 was in 88.2% vascular insufficiency. One-third of the patients suffered from diabetes mellitus.[4]

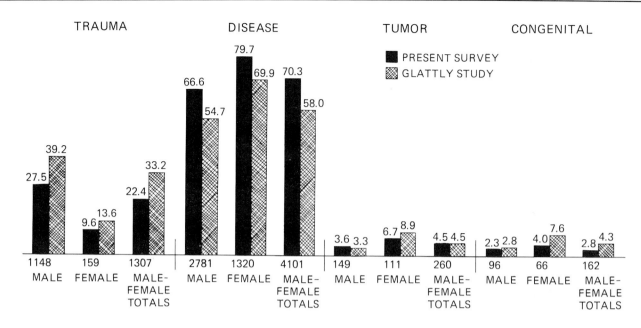

Figure 1-1.   Distribution by cause and sex. (Reprinted by permission from Kay and Newman.[3])

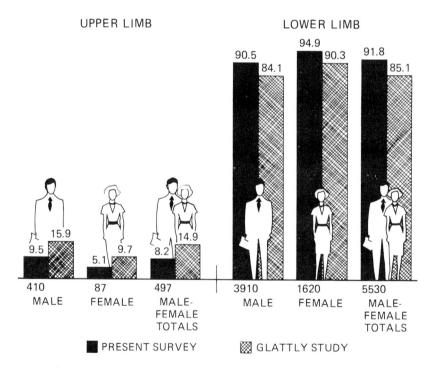

Figure 1-2.   Distribution by extremity and sex. (Reprinted by permission from Kay and Newman.[3])

References

1. Burgess EM, Romano RL: The management of lower extremity amputees using immediate post surgical prostheses. *Clin Orthop* 57:137–146, 1968.

2. Glattly HW: A statistical study of 12,000 new amputees. *South Med J* 57:1373–1378, 1964.

3. Kay HW, Newman JD: Relative incidences of new amputations. *Orthotics and Prosthetics* 29:3–16, 1975.

4. Ebskov B: Choice of level in lower extremity amputation—nationwide survey. Danish Amputation Register, Copenhagen. *Prosthetics and Orthotics Int* 7:58–60, 1983.

CHAPTER 2
Determination of Amputation Levels

Once the decision has been made to amputate, the exact level of amputation must be determined. Several factors influence the decision. The first consideration concerns the personality, sex, age, and occupation of the patient. Closely tied to this is consideration of the prosthetic replacement. The lowest possible level of amputation should be utilized. The older the patient, the more desirable is the creation of an end-bearing stump. In addition, preservation of functioning joints in the amputated extremity is very desirable. In the lower extremity, preservation of the knee joint aids in saving energy for the patient and improves the chances for rehabilitation. Active and unaided ambulation, in turn, improves the long-term prognosis for the patient.

Another factor is the extent of the surgeon's knowledge of basic surgical procedures in amputation surgery. Building on this knowledge, the surgeon may be able to use atypical flaps to cover the stump end and thereby preserve a longer portion of the limb and another joint for the patient.

Paramount in considering the level of amputation is the disease process itself. In the case of a malignant tumor, the choice is clear: The amputation has to be done outside the limits of the malignancy. The same is true for overwhelming infection. Here, too, the amputation must eliminate the disease process outside of its most proximal extent.

The situation is somewhat similar in the patient with acute arterial obstruction. If it is impossible to render the obstructed segment of the blood vessel patent or to bypass it by collateral circulation, the products of the necrotic process will reach the general circulation. Of particular concern is the possibility of the release of greater amounts of myoglobin from large masses of necrotic muscles. Myoglobinuria and eventual renal failure are the possible late results.

As the signs of systemic toxicity increase and the renal function decreases, amputation becomes an emergency procedure. Unfortunately, there are few clinical signs that are helpful in determining the level of amputation. An arteriogram and determination of the skin sensation may be the only preoperative indicators. Otherwise, the final decision has to be made at the time of surgery, when the viability of the tissues can be evaluated by gross inspection. An amputation may have to be carried out more proximally than initially planned, depending on the viability of the tissues.

In patients with chronic vascular insufficiency, a more complex problem arises. Skin changes such as gangrene and ulceration are only the grossly visible expressions of the disease. Most of the time, the entire extremity is involved in the disease process, which leads to occlusion of the blood supply. Amputation proximal to the ulcer or the gangrenous part of the extremity may eliminate the visible disease process. However, the vascular insufficiency further proximally may lead to delayed wound healing or wound breakdown later on, which may, in the end, require revision of the amputation or reamputation at a higher level. Since viable skin remains the most important structure for healing of the amputation wound, most procedures devised to evaluate circulation of the vascular-insufficient extremity concentrate on the competence of the skin circulation, because the absence of a peripheral pulse does not necessarily indicate that the distal part of the extremity is no longer viable. The demand for such a procedure is again the realization that the lower the amputation, the better the chances for the rehabilitation of the patient, while at the same time the patient is spared further procedures to revise a failed amputation.

Examination of the patient with vascular insufficiency should include an arteriogram of the affected extremity. The arteriogram itself does not determine the level of amputation. However, it does give an insight into the anatomic conditions of the vascular tree in the extremity.

Attempts to determine the adequacy of the circulation in the extremity can be divided into invasive and noninvasive procedures. Invasive procedures measure the speed with which an intradermally injected bolus of radioactive material is cleared. Moore[1,2] uses a gamma camera for determination of xenon-133 clearance. The patient is placed in a supine position and allowed to reach equilibrium with room temperature for 15 minutes. The room temperature itself is regulated between 22 to 27°C. Then 100 to 500 μCi of xenon-133 are dissolved in 0.05 ml of saline and injected intradermally with a 26-gauge needle. The site of injection is medially and laterally to the midpoint of the anterior portion of the proposed skin incision. If so desired, the proposed site of the next lower amputation level can be examined at the same time. The xenon activity is monitored for 10 minutes at four frames per minute by the gamma camera and displayed. Blood flow is calculated using the Fick flow equation:

$$F = \frac{100 \times \lambda \times K}{P}$$

where F is skin blood flow in milliliters per 100 g of tissue per minute. K is the flow constant of xenon-133. λ equals the blood per skin coefficient for xenon-133 (0.7). P equals the specific gravity of skin (1.05).

Moore found the minimum acceptable xenon skin blood flow for successful amputation healing to be 1.6 ml per 100 g of tissue per minute.

Measurements of skin perfusion pressure were carried out by Holstein,[3,4] where an intradermally injected dose of iodine-131 or iodine-125 mixed with histamine is put under pressure with a pneumatic tourniquet. The pressure required to stop the washout of the radioactive material from the skin was considered to be the skin perfusion pressure. Where skin perfusion pressure was above 30 mm Hg, 90% of the amputation wounds healed.

An interesting invasive technique is the measurement of the deep muscle temperature in the ischemic limbs, and then correlating them to the successful healing of the amputation wound.[5] In this method, serial temperature measurements are performed in the ischemic limb with a thermistor probe at two levels: 15 cm above and 10 cm below the knee joint space. The measurements start at the subcutaneous level and proceed toward the center of the bone. The difference between the maximum deep muscle temperature at 15 cm above the knee and 10 cm below the knee is called ΔT_{max}. The lower this difference is, the more likely healing in the below-knee amputation will occur. Indeed, where ΔT_{max} is 1.5 C or less, the likelihood of healing in a below-knee amputation is the highest.

Among the noninvasive techniques, the measuring of systolic blood pressure by Doppler ultrasound is probably most commonly used.[6-10] It requires a continuous-wave Doppler ultrasonic velocity detector with the transmission frequency of 5 or 10 MHz and a pneumatic tourniquet of adequate size. The cuff is slowly inflated until the Doppler signal from the peripheral artery disappears. The cuff is then deflated slowly until the signal reappears. A pressure of 70 mm Hg seems to be the critical level for healing.

Another noninvasive technique measures the reflection of a laser beam by moving red blood cells.[11,12] In an experiment, the difference in blood flow down to 1.5 mm from the surface of the skin was measured after inducing varying degrees of erythema with ultraviolet (UV) light. The Doppler shift of laser light backscattered from moving red blood cells in the cutaneous microcirculation was measured. This technique was compared to the xenon clearance technique. Statistical analysis showed that both measurements agreed favorably.

The most promising and, at present, probably the most accurate method of predicting success in major amputations is the transcutaneous measurement of oxygen tension.[13-15] This method has the advantage of a noninvasive procedure and is relatively simple to perform. It is independent from the compressibility of the larger vessels, and it takes into account the impaired oxygen effusion due to the impairment of small vessels. Oxygen sensors, although fairly expensive, are commercially available and accurate. The sensor is calibrated for temperature and atmospheric pressure. It is then applied to the skin, which is heated to 45°C. The sensor stabilizes after approximately 20 minutes. The minimum desirable oxygen tension differs in various studies between 30 to 50 mm Hg. In limbs with vascular insufficiency, there seems to be a gradient with decreasing oxygen tension towards the distal end of the extremity. Another interesting finding is that in some patients with vascular insufficiency of the lower extremities, the oxygen tension is dependent upon the position of the patient: In supine position, the oxygen tension in the lower extremities is lower than with the trunk vertical and the lower extremities horizontal.[13] The measurement of oxygen tension may also give the surgeon the possibility of mapping out areas of greater and lesser perfusion in the involved extremity.

References

1. Malone JM, Leal JM, Moore WS, et al: The "gold standard" for amputation level selection: Xenon-133 clearance. *J Surg Res* 30:449–455, 1981.

2. Moore WS: Determination of amputation level. *Arch Surg* 107:798–802, 1973.

3. Holstein P, Sager P, Lassen NA: Wound healing in below-knee amputations in relation to skin perfusion pressure. *Acta Orthopaedics Scand* 50:49–58, 1979.

4. Holstein P, Dovey H, Lassen NA: Wound healing in above-knee amputations in relation to skin perfusion pressure. *Acta Orthopaedics Scand* 50:59–66, 1979

5. Williams DB, Karl RC: Measurement of deep muscle temperature in ischemic limbs. *A J Surg* 139:503–507, April 1980.

6. Barnes RW, Shanik GD, Slaymaker EE: An index of healing in below-knee amputation: Leg blood pressure by Doppler ultrasound. *Surgery* 79(1):13–20, 1976.

7. Creaney MG, Chattopadhaya DK, Ward AS, Morris-Jones W: Doppler ultrasound in the assessment of amputation level. *J Royal Coll Surg (Edinburgh)* 26:278–281, 1981.

8. Dean RH, Yao JST, Thompson RG, et al: Predictive value of ultrasonically derived arterial pressure in determination of amputation level. *Am Surg* 41(11):731–737, 1975.

9. Nicholas GG, Myers JL, DeMuth WE Jr: The role of vascular laboratory criteria in the selection of patients for lower extremity amputation. *Ann Surg* 195(4):469–473, 1982.

10. Cederberg PA, Pritchard JJ, Hoyce JW: Doppler-determined segmental pressures and wound healing in amputations for vascular disease. *J Bone Joint Surg* 65-A:363–365, 1983.

11. Holloway GA Jr, Watkins DW: Laser Doppler measurement of cutaneous blood flow. *J Invest Dermatol* 69(1):306–309, 1977.

12. Holloway GA Jr, Burgess EM: Preliminary experiences with laser Doppler velocimetry for the determination of amputation levels. Center for Bioengineering, University of Washington, Seattle. *Prosthetics and Orthotics Int* 7:63–60, 1983.

13. Burgess EM, Matsen FA, Wyss CR, et al: Segmental transcutaneous measurements of Po_2 in patients requiring below-the-knee amputation for peripheral vascular insufficiency. *J Bone Joint Surg* 64-A:378–382, 1982.

14. Christensen SK, Klarke M: Transcutaneous oxygen measurement in peripheral occlusive disease — An indicator of wound healing in leg amputation. *J Bone Joint Surg* 68-B:423–426, 1986.

15. Katsamouris A, Brewster DC, Megerman J, et al: Transcutaneous oxygen-tension in selection of amputation level. *Am J Surg* 147:510–517, 1984.

CHAPTER 3
Pediatric Considerations

Although there is no great difference in surgical techniques for amputations performed on children compared with those done on adults, the factors of continuing growth and anatomic differences do require some modification of the principles.

No ideal level of amputation can be stated as a definitive rule. However, in the child even more than in the adult, conservation of as much length as possible is desirable. In particular, disarticulation and preservation of the adjacent epiphysis is vastly preferable to an amputation through the metaphysis or diaphysis. On the other hand, preservation of the knee, elbow, or wrist joint is preferable to performing a disarticulation in the next higher joint.

The skin and subcutaneous tissue of a child are more likely to withstand tight closure. Also, thick split thickness skin grafts are much more likely to provide permanent skin coverage than in the adult; in children, they withstand the pressure from prostheses surprisingly well.

Soft tissue coverage of the bony stump and maintenance of a distal insertion of the transected muscle should be provided by myoplasty rather than myodesis in the child. The latter requires injury to the distal end of the bony stump and may enhance the overgrowth of the bone. This bony overgrowth, which occurs to a much lesser extent in the adult, is due to appositional accretion of osseous tissue at the distal end of the bony stump, rather than a vis a tergo from the epiphysis at the proximal end of the amputated bone. It leads to a spike-like structure of ever increasing length that, if unchecked, may perforate the overlying soft tissues including the skin, leading to an infection. Various procedures have been recommended to counteract this overgrowth, including both the capping of the exposed marrow cavity with a silastic plug and osteoplastic treatment of the bone end by coverage with an osteoperiosteal flap, or the formation of a bony bridge between tibia and fibula by osteoperiosteal flaps in the below-knee amputation.

All transected nerves develop neuromas. Amputation neuromas in the child often grow to grotesque sizes. However, unless they are in an area of direct pressure and subject to traction and tension in scar tissue, they are rarely the cause of discomfort. Phantom sensation is very likely to be present in any child with an acquired amputation. It seems, however, that the sensation is less bothersome in children than adults; and the younger the child is at the time of the amputation, the more vague the recollection of the phantom sensation later on. Beyond the age of 10 years, all children complain of phantom limb sensation following amputation. Phantom pain, however, is rarely a complaint in a child amputee.

CHAPTER *4*
Preoperative Considerations

POSITIONING

For most of the procedures in amputation surgery, the patient should be kept in a supine position. Only procedures close to the trunk, such as disarticulation of the hip and shoulder and forequarter and hindquarter amputations, may require side positioning of the patient. On occasion, the side position may also prove more comfortable if an above-knee amputation is necessary in the case of a knee fusion. The prone position may be the position of choice in the case of below-knee amputation in the patient with limited motion or fusion of the hip.

TOURNIQUETS

Most of the amputations of the distal parts of the extremities are done under tourniquet control. The tourniquet can be maintained in the sterile field as long as it is adequately sterilized. The pneumatic tourniquet is preferable to others, since its pressure can be controlled with a manometer. However, an adequately sterilized elastic bandage, such as an Esmarch of adequate width, is sure to give satisfactory hemostasis if it is applied with sufficient tension. A special method of tourniquet control is the application of an Esmarch bandage through the perineum over a Steinmann pin inserted through the soft tissue above the greater trochanter. This maneuver allows hemostasis for at least a short period of time in cases of high above-knee amputations.

The use of a tourniquet in patients with vascular insufficiency is usually not necessary; in fact, it is discouraged because of the lack of oxygen in the tissues of the extremity to be amputated. It is, however, recommended to put a tourniquet on the extremity, even if it is not inflated, to guard against sudden unsuspected hemorrhage.

Whenever used, the tourniquet should be released prior to wound closure to ensure meticulous hemostasis. The reactive hyperemia usually shows the blood vessels that need attention.

CLEANSING

Preparation of the extremity to be amputated starts with the shaving of the area to be exposed as the operative field. A thorough cleansing of the extremity with soap and water prior to surgery is desirable. The final preparation of the extremity is done with bacteriacidal solution such as Betadine (povidone-iodine), or a mercury derivative.

DRAPING

Free draping of the extremity to be amputated is essential, since the ablated part of the extremity ultimately has to be handed off the table. However, the distal parts of the extremity can be dropped into a sterile sheet without any particular preparation, and thereby draped out of the field. This should be done routinely where an infected part of the distal end of the extremity has to be separated completely from the sterile field. In these cases, plastic sheets with skin adherent are particularly valuable since they provide an airtight enclosure for the part of the extremity they cover.

Draping for the more distal parts of the extremity is best done by providing a cuff of sufficient length, with the drapes over the proximal end of the prepared extremity. This allows adequate, free motion in the more proximal joints, and therefore adequate access to the circumference of the extremity Figures 4–1 through 4–3 depict the simple draping of an extremity. In disarticulations of the hip or the

Figures 4-1 to 4-3.   Simple draping of an extremity.

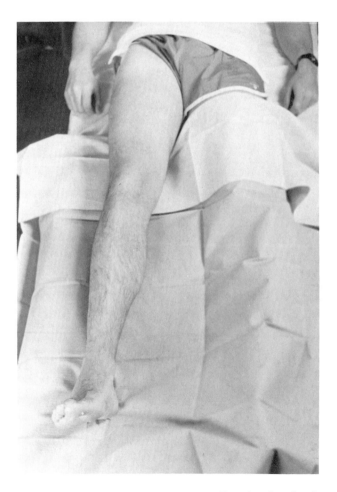

Figure 4-1.   A sheet with an adequate cuff is placed under the lower extremity.

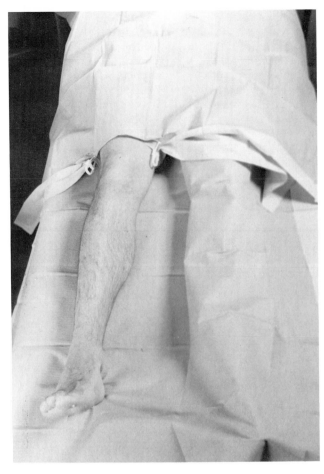

Figure 4-2.   A second sheet is placed over the lower extremity and affixed to the cuff of the first sheet with towel clips.

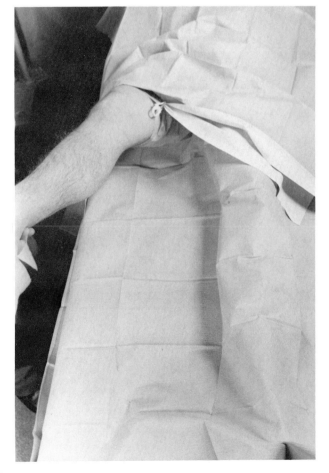

Figure 4-3.   This arrangement allows reasonable mobility of the extremity.

shoulder, a triangle or a square has to be formed out of three or four drapes to cover an area proximal to the area to be amputated. A similar mechanism of draping possibly with more corners may have to be used in more corpulent patients undergoing fore-quarter or hindquarter amputation. Figures 4–4 through 4–8 show the draping of the shoulder girdle for a proximal humeral amputation or a shoulder disarticulation.

Figures 4-4 to 4-8.   Draping of the shoulder girdle for proximal humeral amputation or shoulder disarticulation.

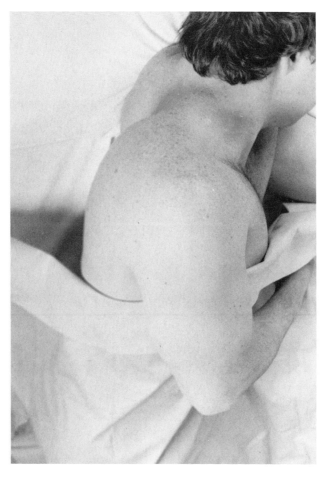

Figure 4-4.   The first sheet is placed under the upper extremity on the chest wall.

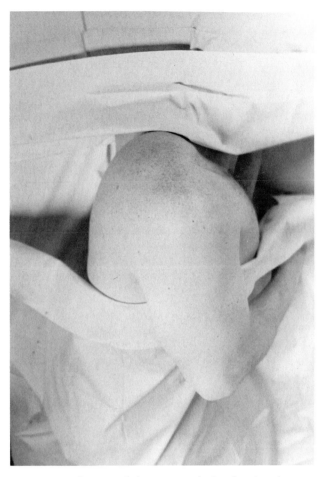

Figure 4-5.   The second sheet covers the head and neck.

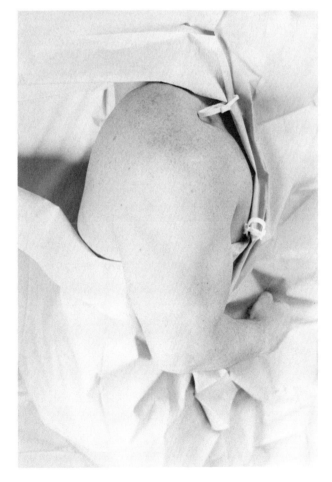

Figure 4-6.   The anterior part of the chest wall is covered.

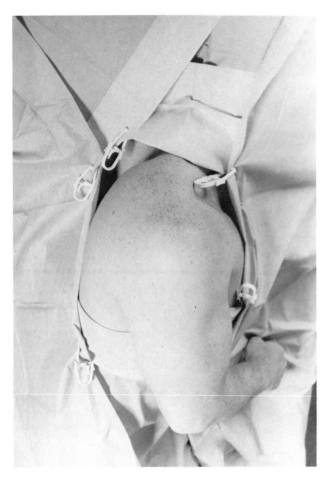

Figure 4-7. Two sheets are used to cover the back of the head and the posterior chest wall.

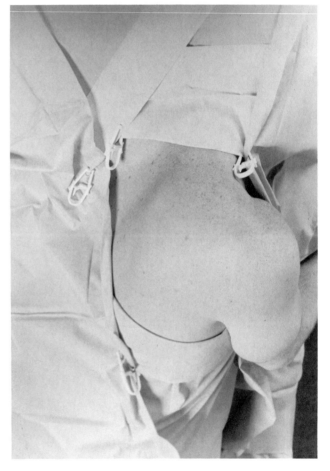

Figure 4-8. The draping with several sheets gives enough mobility to move the patient back and forth to approach the anterior and posteior part of the area of the shoulder girdle.

CHAPTER 5
Anesthesia

Steven F. Seidman

Current standards of anesthetic care dictate the use of the technique (general anesthesia, spinal or epidural block, or peripheral nerve block) that is best suited to the individual patient's physiologic needs, comfort, and psychological well-being, as well as the creation of surgical conditions deemed most suitable for the proposed procedure. For amputation surgery, there is a choice among anesthetic techniques to achieve these goals; in fact, usually there is no absolute indication for choosing one anesthetic technique over the other. The decision usually revolves around relative indications, such as: 1) the preoperative condition of the patient, with particular emphasis on the cardiovascular, respiratory, and central nervous systems; 2) the desires of the patient along with past anesthetic experiences; and 3) the particular preferences and experience of the anesthesiologist and surgeon.

GENERAL ANESTHESIA

When faced with the loss of a limb, virtually all oriented patients will choose general anesthesia over modalities with which they would feel no pain but would be aware that an amputation was being performed. Furthermore, the depth of general anesthesia is easily adjusted so that the technique does not need to be abandoned if there is insufficient analgesia and reflex movement.

General anesthesia also proves advantageous when the dissection proceeds more proximally than was initially expected. In such a case, a peripheral nerve block may be insufficient. Tourniquet pain is not a problem under general anesthesia, although the inflation of the tourniquet may produce activa-

tion of the sympathetic nervous system with resultant hypertension and tachycardia.

The use of general anesthesia has some drawbacks as well as advantages. General anesthesia for the patient about to undergo an amputation can be accomplished by a narcotic technique, or by the use of halogenated hydrocarbons (e.g., Halothane, Ethrane®, or Forane®), or by a combination of both techniques. Narcotics are supplemented with nitrous oxide, sedatives such as droperiodol or diazepam, and muscle relaxants. For amputations, volatile halogenated hydrocarbons are usually supplemented with nitrous oxide and, sometimes, with narcotics. The narcotic technique has, as its major drawback, significant respiratory depression that may extend into the postoperative period, especially if it is insufficiently reversed. The narcotic technique causes less cardiovascular depression than halogenated hydrocarbons, although hypotension may result in a patient with insufficient volume replacement. The major disadvantage of the narcotic technique involves activation of the sympathetic nervous system, especially after incisional, tourniquet, or periosteal pain. This activation results in hypertension and tachycardia if the level of anesthesia is not deep enough. The use of volatile halogenated hydrocarbons is associated with respiratory and cardiovascular depression. These agents are more effective than narcotics in protecting against activation of the sympathetic nervous system, in that the depth of anesthesia is easily and rapidly controllable. Unlike narcotics, however, halogenated hydrocarbons provide little postoperative analgesia. On this basis, one might consider infiltration of long acting local anesthetics (e.g., Marcaine®) in the vicinity of exposed nerves after amputation when using general anesthesia.

To understand the potential problems of general anesthesia in amputation surgery, one must consider the patient population. In the otherwise healthy patient, amputation surgery for a congenital anomaly, tumor, or trauma may be performed with the patient tolerating the physiologic insults induced by general anesthesia quite well. However, amputations are often performed in patients with pre-existing medical problems. Included in this category are: 1) patients with peripheral vascular disease associated with either generalized, atherosclerotic cardiovascular disease, and/or diabetes mellitus; 2) patients with generalized or localized sepsis; and 3) patients with chemical or electrical injuries or trauma to multiple organ systems. Patients with generalized atherosclerosis often have coronary artery disease and systemic hypertension. Tachycardia and added hypertension induced by surgical stimulation or tourniquet inflation may induce myocardial decompensation. This decompensation can be compounded by myocardial depression induced by halogenated hydrocarbons. In the same patient group, cerebral vascular accidents are common. This possibility may be enhanced by the added hypertension induced by surgical stimulation or tourniquet inflation. Patients with diabetes mellitus may have preexisting renal dysfunction, which can prolong the excretion of the anesthetic agents. Patients with thermal, chemical, or electrical injuries or who are in post-traumatic states, and those with smoke inhalation, toxic gas inhalation, or chest wall injury, may have a pre-existing respiratory dysfunction that can be accentuated under general anesthesia with resultant decreased functional residual capacity, ventilation-perfusion mismatching, and atelectasis.

SPINAL OR EPIDURAL ANESTHESIA

Both spinal and epidural anesthesia induce surgical analgesia for amputations involving the lower extremity. The appropriate use of amnestic supplements (e.g., diazepam) can produce virtually total amnesia regarding the surgical procedure. Spinal anesthesia yields a more complete and dependable sensory block than does epidural anesthesia. A major advantage of the epidural approach, however, is that a teflon catheter can be inserted into the epidural space, and multiple supplements to the local anesthesia can be injected through this catheter. This continuous technique allows intraoperative adjustment of the height of the block and its intensity and duration. Although a catheter may also be inserted into the subarachnoid space to achieve continuous spinal anesthesia, the risks of infection and the associated disastrous consequences are too high. Therefore, spinal anesthesia is a "one-shot" procedure. If the anesthesia begins to wear off, either the spinal block must be performed again or, as is usually the case, the anesthesiologist must resort to general anesthesia. On the other hand, if a continuous epidural anesthesia begins to fail, injection of additional local anesthetic will serve as a reinforcement.

In amputations of the lower extremity, the level to which the spinal or epidural anesthesia block must extend cephalad is crucial for the success of the analgesia. According to Murphy,[1] the sympathetic nervous system contains not only visceral efferent fibers, but also afferent sensory fibers. These afferent fibers travel along with the sympathetic nerves, and then via the sympathetic trunk and white rami communicantes to the neuraxis; and they may enter the spinal cord at a level higher than that predicted by traditional dermatomal patterns. An example serves to illustrate this situation. A foot amputation may be performed under a spinal or epidural block that extends no higher than L3. If one uses a thigh tourniquet, however, the pain generated after tourniquet inflation may travel with sympathetic afferent fibers that enter the spinal cord at considerably higher levels. Observing the traditional dermatomal pattern, a block to the level of L2 should prevent pain perception associated with tourniquet inflation. Apparently, however, there are afferent fibers that trasmit pressure sensations that enter the cord at levels considerably cephalad to L2.

Thus, if the spinal or epidural block extends only to L2, the patient will complain of tourniquet pain. The block must extend to a level of T10 for satisfactory analgesia after tourniquet inflation.

Assuming that the spinal or epidural block extends no higher than T10, the cardiovascular derangements associated with these blocks can usually be easily managed. Both types of blocks will induce a drop in blood pressure due to a decrease in sympathetic tone. The decrease in blood pressure occurs more abruptly with spinal than epidural blockage. Such hypotension can be managed with volume infusion and if necessary with vasopressors. Because of the possibility of inducing hypotension with these blocks, their use in the face of marginal cardiovascular function and/or decreased circulating blood volume (e.g., hemorrhagic shock after trauma) should be undertaken only with extreme caution. An advantage of both blocks is that they cause minimal derangement of respiratory functions, assuming that the level does not become too cephalad. Neither a spinal nor epidural block should be attempted if there is any suspicion that the patient has a coagulopathy such as disseminated intravascular coagulation. This coagulopathy may be associated with trauma and burn injuries,[2] and a subarachnoid and/or epidural hematoma might result if either block is attempted. Any pre-existing or concurrent coagulopathy is a contraindication to an attempted spinal or epidural block. The presence of peripheral or central nervous system disease may represent relative contraindications to such blocks. Under no circumstances should a spinal or epidural block be attempted if there is any sign or suspicion of infection involving the tissue in the vicinity of the prospective needle insertion.

PERIPHERAL NERVE BLOCKS

Peripheral nerve blocks and intravascular regional blocks provide a multitude of advantages over general, spinal, or epidural anesthesia. Although peripheral blocks are devoid of any amnestic properties, they provide excellent analgesia, since all afferent impulses are blocked. These blocks offer effective postoperative analgesia, assuming long-acting local anesthetics have been used. Peripheral nerve blocks involve no respiratory or cardiovascular derangements; as a result, they are excellent choices for the patient with pre-existing pulmonary or cardiac disease. Also, if an amputation must be performed on an emergency basis on a patient who has recently eaten, a nerve block yields adequate analgesia without causing loss of consciousness or loss of the protective laryngeal reflexes. As a result, aspiration pneumonitis should not prove to be a complication. In patients with pre-existing medical conditions in whom a peripheral nerve block is contemplated, the anesthesiologist can assure the patient of virtually complete amnesia, if so desired, through the judicious use of sedatives.

Peripheral nerve blocks should not be employed in close proximity to an infected area. Although not indicated in patients who are fully anticoagulated, the use of peripheral nerve blocks in patient receiving so-called "miniheparin" remains a debated issue. Nerve blocks are often time-consuming and technically difficult for those who perform them infrequently; and they are not as reliable in inducing analgesia as general, spinal, or epidural anesthesia. For this reason, many surgeons and anesthesiologists avoid peripheral nerve blocks in amputative surgery. Intravascular regional blocks are more reliable and require less technical expertise.

Major complications of peripheral nerve blocks include toxic overdoses of local anesthetic after both inadvertent intravascular injection and potential nerve damage subsequent either to the injected local anesthetic itself or to unsuspected injection into the nerve substance. Peripheral nerve blocks involving the upper extremity carry the risk of pneumothorax, potential nerve block involving the vagus, phrenic, or recurrent laryngeal nerve, and inadvertent injection into the subarachnoid or epidural space. The major complication after an intravascular regional block centers around tourniquet failure, with the subsequent introduction of a potentially toxic overdose of local anesthetic into the systemic circulation.

Amputations involving the upper extremity are well handled with some form of brachial plexus block. The brachial plexus is usually approached via the axillary, supraclavicular, or interscalene approach. The infraclavicular approach as described by Raj et al.[3] is not frequently employed. These techniques will not be described in detail in this chapter, and the reader is referred to the excellent descriptions of the mechanics of these blocks by Moore[4] and Winnie.[5] It should be noted that with regard to pe-

ripheral nerve blocks, Lofstrom et al. have reported a correlation between the number of injections and complications such as postinjection neuropathy and intravascular injections.[6] Thus, a well-placed peripheral nerve block involving a minimum number of injections should minimize the chances of a toxic overdose of local anesthetic and of a postinjection neuropathy. With the axillary, supraclavicular, and interscalene approaches, the anesthesiologist must separately block the intercostobrachial nerve, which is the lateral branch of the T2 intercostal nerve, if a tourniquet is to be used.[1,4] This nerve, which innervates the medial border of the upper arm and (to a variable extent) the skin in the axilla, is easily blocked with a cuff of anesthesia over the medial aspect of the upper arm.

Each of these approaches has its own advantages and disadvantages. The axillary approach according to Murphy[1] is the preferred technique of regional anesthesia for surgical procedures distal to the elbow. According to Moore, this approach may be used for upper arm surgery if one has also blocked the medial brachial cutaneous nerve, the intercostobrachial nerve, the superficial cervical plexus, or all three.[4] The axillary approach makes it virtually impossible to block the phrenic, vagus, or recurrent laryngeal nerves inadvertently. Pneumothorax, subarachnoid, or epidural injection and stellate ganglion block would also be most unusual with this approach. This technique cannot be used, however, when the patient cannot sufficiently abduct the arm to expose the axilla. Intravenous injection of a local anesthetic with consequent toxic overdoses may occur. The axillary approach may require separate blocking of the musculocutaneous nerve within the coracobrachialis muscle in the axilla if insufficient volumes of local anesthetic are initially used. Otherwise, the lateral aspect of the forearm may remain unanesthetized. Winnie points out that the axillary approach is contraindicated with infection or malignancy in the involved extremity, and that this block is difficult to perform in an obese individual and in those in whom the axillary artery is not palpable.[7]

The supraclavicular approach to the brachial plexus, as opposed to the axillary approach, produces anesthesia of the upper extremity even when: 1) the arm cannot be abducted; 2) the surgery or manipulation involves either the shoulder, girdle or axilla; or 3) if there is an infection of the arm. Contraindications to the supraclavicular approach include the lack of patient cooperation and concurrent respiratory dysfunction. The frequency of occurrence of penumothorax after an attempted supraclavicular block has been reported by Moore[4] to be 0.5 to 5%. This frequency decreases with increasing experience and skill on the anesthesiologist's part, and seems to be highest in tall, thin patients. The first indication of penumothorax is chest pain, usually exacerbated by deep breathing. Chest pain my not be reported until 12 hours after the block has been attempted; for this reason, patients should be observed for up to 24 hours after the supraclavicular injection. Other complications of this approach include phrenic nerve block, which may occur in 40 to 60% of cases. Given the incidence of penumothoraces and phrenic nerve block after supraclavicular approaches, this block should not be performed bilaterally in patients with underlying pulmonary disease (e.g., emphysema), nor in those who have sustained chest trauma. Other complications include stellate ganglion block and, rarely, subarachnoid injections or toxic reactions due to inadvertent intravascular injections. The supraclavicular brachial plexus block does not produce analgesia after tourniquet inflation. As with the axillary approach, the intercostobrachial nerve must be blocked with a cuff of local anesthesia around the inner aspect of the proximal arm.

The interscalene approach to the brachial plexus block has been described by Winnie.[7] Most of the space between the anterior and middle scalene muscles lies above the cupola of the lung and the subclavian artery; from this standpoint, the interscalene approach allows for greater safety than the supraclavicular approach. Occasionally, blockade of the ulnar nerve is either absent or insufficient after an interscalene injection. Analgesia in the distribution of the ulnar nerve must be assessed prior to any amputation involving this distribution. If insufficient ulnar analgesia is present, a separate block of the ulnar nerve is necessary. If a tourniquet is to be used, the intercostobrachial nerve must be blocked separately. The interscalene approach is suggested by Winnie in upper extremity procedures on: 1) obese patients in whom an axillary or supraclavicular approach may be technically quite difficult; and 2) on children or intoxicated individuals from whom one cannot expect much cooperation. Surgery about the shoulder girdle and upper arm may be performed under interscalene block, and infection and/or malignancy in the arm does not present contraindications to its use. It is rare to cause a pneumothorax during an interscalene block. Drawbacks to the interscalene approach include: 1) the slow onset and often inadequate analgesia of the ulnar nerve; 2) possible vertebral artery injection; and 3) inadvertant placement of the local anesthetic into the subarachnoid or epidural space. Other possible complications include phrenic, vagus, and recurrent laryngeal nerve blockade; for this reason, bilateral interscalene blocks should not be attempted to avoid the possibility of respiratory decompensation.[7] A one-sided interscalene block may be used even in the patient with pre-existing respiratory dysfunction.

The use of peripheral nerve blocks for amputations or other surgical procedures involving the lower extremity has prompted much debate. Bridenbaugh has pointed out that for surgery involving the lower leg or foot, a peripheral nerve block is the method of choice. Moore claims that lower extremity surgery above the knee necessitates the use not only of sciatic and femoral nerve blocks, but also of lateral femoral cutaneous and obturator nerve blocks. Since obturator nerve blocks are often unsuccessful, Moore suggests using spinal or epidural anesthesia in those patients in whom regional anesthesia is desired. An alternative has been described by Winnie, wherein anesthesia for the entire leg may be provided with a combination of sciatic and femoral nerve blocks — the so-called "3-in-1" block.[8] This block involves some modification of the usual techniques for femoral nerve block. An increased volume of local anesthetic is injected after eliciting femoral nerve paresthesia. This technique of Winnie's — also known as the inguinal paravascular technique — allows a block of the obturator, the lateral femoral cutaneous, and the femoral nerve with one injection. Multiple techniques have been described regarding sciatic nerve blocks, and the reader is referred to any of the standard texts on nerve blocks. It should be repeated, however, that anesthesia for the entire leg requires the use of femoral, obturator, lateral femoral cutaneous, and sciatic nerve blocks. Tourniquet inflation in the thigh region would also require that all four of these nerves be blocked. Unlike peripheral nerve blocks for the upper extremity, those for the lower extremity involve few complications other than intravascular injection with resultant systemic toxicity and potential postblock neuropathy. As with upper extremity blocks, nerve blocks of the leg should not be performed in the vicinity of infection or malignancy. Furthermore, if no intravascular injection has taken place, no respiratory or cardiovascular derangements should occur during peripheral nerve blocks of the lower extremity. These blocks also offer postoperative analgesia if long-acting local anesthetics are used.

INTRAVENOUS REGIONAL ANESTHESIA

Surgical procedures on the extremities may also be carried out with intravenous regional anesthesia — a technique called the Bier block. This technique is not commonly used in amputation procedures because of the necessity of exsanguinating the extremity prior to the intravenous injection of the local anesthetic, and of cannulating a vein in the region of the prospective amputation. The necessity for venous cannulation makes this technique unsuitable in the presence of infection or malignancy. Manipulation of an extremity that has had traumatic involvement or that has been subjected to chemical, thermal, or electrical injury is usually not clinically justified. As a result, the indications for intravenous regional anesthesia are markedly limited in amputation surgery. Some of its advantages, however, are its technical simplicity, its virtually guaranteed surgical analgesia, and the usual absence of cardiovascular and respiratory complications. Toxic, systemic responses to the local anesthetics employed with this modality may occur after tourniquet malfunction or after the intentional deflation of the tourniquet. The toxic responses are directly proportional to the dose of the anesthetic; they may be a function of the tourniquet time, and they are generally referable to the cardiovascular and central nervous systems.[9] The total dose of anesthesia required for the intravenous regional technique makes it more suitable for upper extremity rather than lower extremity surgery.

References

1. Murphy TM: Nerve blocks. In Miller R (ed): *Anesthesia.* Churchill Livingstone, 1981, p 642.

2. Ellison N, Joves S: Diagnosis and disorders of hemostasis. *ASA Refresher Courses in Anesthesiology,* vol 7. 1979, p 98.

3. Raj P, et al: Infraclavicular brachial plexus block — A new approach. *Anesth. Analg* 56:554, 1977.

4. Moore D: *Regional Block,* ed 4. Charles C Thomas, Springfield, Ill, 1978.

5. Winnie A: The perivascular techniques of brachial plexus anesthesia. In *ASA Refresher Courses in Anesthesiology,* vol 2. 1974, pp 149–162.

6. Lofstrom B, et al: Late disturbances in nerve function after block with local anesthetic agents — An electro-neurographic study. *Acta Anesth Scand* 10:111, 1966.

7. Winnie A: Regional anesthesia of upper and lower extremities. In Zauder H (ed): *Anesthesia for Orthopaedic Surgery.* FA Davis, 1980, p 94.

8. Winnie A, et al: The Inquinal paravascular technique of lumbar plexus anesthesia: The "3 in 1" block. *Anesth Amalg* 52:989, 1973.

9. Zauder H: Intravenous Regional Anesthesia. In Zauder H (ed): *Anesthesia for Orthopaedic Surgery.* FA Davis, 1980, p 123.

CHAPTER 6
Tissue Management

After the removal of the diseased part of the extremity, the patient is left with a wound of considerable size. Treatment of exposed tissues is crucial for obtaining a well-functioning stump. It is most desirable that the stump be painless, have well-placed minimal scars, and that the bony stump be well covered by soft tissue — preferably active musculature.

SKIN

Coverage of the amputation stump with well-vascularized skin flaps that heal by primary intention remains the most important tissue consideration in amputation surgery. Attempts to predict the perfusion and, therefore, viability of the skin have been mentioned. Beyond that, it has to be understood that some of the blood vessels to the skin will have to be interrupted during surgery. However, keeping undermining of the skin to a minimum and leaving functioning musculature below the skin flaps intact decreases the danger of skin breakdown. Skin closure under tension should be avoided in adults since it too can obstruct skin circulation. In children, snug skin closure does not seem to be as worrisome as in adults. If possible, the scar should be placed in such a way that it does not interfere with the weight-bearing areas in the future prosthesis.

Skin grafting, especially of the lower extremity stump, has been discouraged in the past. However, experience shows that in adults, split thickness grafts can withstand prosthetic wear if they are over soft tissue and not adherent to bone or thick scars.[1] Pedicle grafts do even better as long as they are not in the immediate weight-bearing area of the stump. In children, even extensive skin grafting may be successful.[2]

In adults as well as children, the success of the graft and the survival of the stump depend upon the meticulous care the patient gives to the stump. A skin care program such as that outlined by Rosenfelder[1] has to be taught to the patient (Table 6-1). In this program, there are three principles of skin care:

1. Cleanliness, including the removal of dry skin and crusts.
2. Maintenance of the pliability of the skin.
3. Decrease of the heat and friction in the prosthesis, which surprisingly enough can be done quite effectively by the use of a plastic sandwich bag. (Another more expensive adjunct to decrease the friction in the socket is the use of silastic jelly-filled socket inserts.)

Table 6-1. Skin Care Program for Patients

Before Prosthetic Fitting

1. *Keep skin and dressing clean*
   Wash your stump daily with soap and water. Use an unmedicated, unscented soap unless a special preparation has been prescribed. Change protective dressings as ordered by the physician. If you use an elastic bandage, have several, and wear a clean one each day. Wash, rinse, and dry bandages thoroughly before wearing again.

2. *Remove dry skin and crusts*
   Apply lotion to your stump and work it into the skin gently, giving special attention to flaky or crusted areas. Be careful not to tear any of the crusts; remove only those which slide off easily. Use an unmedicated, unscented lotion, such as Nivea®, unless a special preparation has been prescribed.

3. *Make the skin pliable*
   Hold fingers in one place on the stump and gently move the skin over the underlying tissues using a circular motion. Pick up the fingers and repeat in an adjacent area. Repeat until the entire grafted or scarred area has been treated. Work *toward* scars to avoid spreading them. In the same way, work *toward* areas where the skin is tight, such as over the end of the stump. You should carry out step 2 and step 3 twice daily—after your bath and at one other time.

After Prosthetic Fitting

1. Continue step 2 and step 3 (above) each day after your bath.

2. Reduce heat and moisture in the socket. Wear a plastic sandwich bag under your stump sock whenever you wear your prosthesis. Check several times a day because the plastic bag may break, and its effectiveness will be lost.

MUSCLE

Under normal circumstances, the skeletal muscles provide active motion in the joints they span. They balance the load upon the neighboring bones and, lastly, help in the fluid transport through their contractions. When a muscle loses one of its points of attachment, it contracts and atrophies. Therefore, attempts should be made during the amputation to counteract the resting tension in the muscle and maintain its length. It is desirable to give a muscle a new distal attachment against which it can work in isometric and isotonic contractions. Myodesis provides an attachment by suturing the severed muscle to the distal end of the bony stump, and then anchoring the sutures in drill holes at the stump end. Myoplasty attempts the same by suturing the beveled-cut surface of one muscle group to its antagonist or the periosteum of the cut bone. In either case, it is highly desirable to avoid lifting the enveloping fascia from the underlying muscle since it is very easily subject to necrosis.

Mondry[3] has recommended that in the above-knee amputation, a two-layer myoplasty be carried out. The deep layer combines the free end of the adductor muscle with the iliotibial tract and vastus lateralis. The more superficial muscle layer combines knee flexors and extensors.

Large areas of necrotic muscle that are commonly found in limbs with vascular insufficiency should be excised. The viable muscles should be handled as delicately and as little as possible to avoid further necrosis.

BONES

It has been a goal for years to create a stump that is able to withstand axial stresses. In the lower extremity amputee, this would mean an end-bearing stump. Only in the partial foot amputation, the Syme amputation, and the knee disarticulation can this goal be realized. Usually the transected end of the bone is too tender to bear weight. In the prosthesis, therefore, the weight-bearing area is shifted away from the stump end to a more proximal, less sensitive location, and the stump is used as a piston that powers the prosthesis.

The idea of turning the cut bone into a closed unit again led to the development of the osteoplastic closure of the open marrow cavity. It was first conceived at the end of the 19th century and was reintroduced during and after the World War II. In the below-knee amputation, the procedure consists of a somewhat longer osteoperiosteal flap from the fibula and two flaps from the tibia to connect the two bones in the lower leg, thus forming a firm osseous bridge between them.[3,4]

NERVES

Transection of the nerves during amputation leads without exception to the formation of a so-called amputation neuroma. A great majority of these amputation neuromas are painless or cause only minimal discomfort under sustained and severe compression. There are, however, patients with painful neuromas that require revision and, on occasion, special procedures.

During amputation, each nerve should be identified, dissected free to a level well above amputation, ligated where concomitant vessels are expected, and cut under minimal tension. The cut end ideally is located in a soft tissue bed, where good circulation surrounds it and where it is not likely to be involved in the scar formation at the stump end. When the amputation neuroma is caught in the scar tissue, it can become a problem that may require both revision and resection of the neuroma and one of the adjuvant procedures.

Of these adjuvant procedures, silicone capping is the most promising.[5] A 5-0 nonabsorbable suture is passed through the closed end of a silicone cap and continued as a Bunnell-type suture through the nerve proximally to the neuroma. The neuroma itself is then resected, and the silicone cap is guided over the free end of the Bunnell suture onto the cut end of the nerve. The open lumen of the silicone cap has to be slightly larger than the diameter of the nerve, and the cap itself should be 5 to 10 times the diameter of the nerve in length. It is either allowed to retract with the nerve end into the soft tissue or, where adequate soft tissue is lacking, a transcutaneous absorbable suture is used to fix the cap in an area where heavy pressure is not expected. Thus, the formation of bulbous neuromas can be prevented.

Another method of dealing with painful neuromas is the implantation of the nerve ending into the medullary cavity of the bone.[6,7] Either 4 or 5 cm of the painful nerve have to be dissected free. Two holes are drilled into the adjacent long bone. The proximal hole is slightly larger than the nerve itself. The distal hole is 1.5 cm away from the first and is slightly smaller. The neuroma is then resected and a 2-0 or 3-0 nonabsorbable suture is passed through the free end of the nerve. This suture is then passed into the first and out of the second hole. Along with the suture, the free end of the nerve is led into the marrow cavity. The end of the suture is secured with a silver clip and bone wax outside of the second hole.

Other methods of dealing with painful neuromas have been described, such as end-to-end anatomosis of two groups of cut fascicles[8] and multiple ligatures of the nerve ends.[9]

In the first method, the painful neuroma is resected, the exposed fascicles of the nerve are divided into two equal bundles, and—using a microsurgical technique—an end-to-end anastomosis of the free ends of the two bundles is accomplished.

In the second technique, the painful neuroma and the adjacent end of the nerve are exposed. The neuroma is resected, and four ligatures are placed around the end of the stump in 5 mm intervals. These ligatures should not be so tight as to crush the nerve, but just snuggly encompass its circumference.

BLOOD VESSELS

The larger veins and arteries must be dissected, and doubly ligated before transection. It is advisable not to catch neighboring veins and arteries in the same ligature; it is indeed better to ligate and section veins and arteries at different levels to avoid the development of aneurysms.

Smaller vessels can be cauterized. Good hemostasis is desirable. Drainage of the wound bed for the first 24 to 48 hours is a rule.

References

1. Rosenfelder R: The below knee amputee with skin grafts. *Phys Ther* 50:1338–1346, 1970.
2. Thomson HG, Martin SR, Murray JF: Skin-grafted juvenile amputation stumps. Are they durable? *Plast Reconstr Surg* 65:195–198, 1980.
3. Mondry F: Der muskelkräftige Ober-und Unterschenkelstumpf. *Der Chirurg* 23:517–519, 1952.
4. Ertl J: Über Amputationsstümpfe. *Der Chirurg* 20:218–224, 1949.
5. Swanson AB, Boeve NR, Lumsden RM: The prevention and treatment of amputation neuromata by silicone capping. *J Hand Surg* 2:70–78, 1977.
6. Boldrey E: Amputation neuroma in nerves, implanted in bone. *Ann Surg* 118:1052–1057, 1943.
7. Hemmy DC: Intramedullary implantation in amputation and other traumatic neuromas. *J Neurosurg* 54:842–843, 1981.
8. Slooff ACJ: Microsurgical possibilities in the treatment of peripheral pain. *Clin Neurol Neurosurg* 80:107–111, 1980.
9. Lengenhager K: Genese und Therapie der Kausalgie. *Hel Chir Acta* 39:685–690, 1972.

Chapter 7
Postoperative Care

Postoperative care of the amputee has two main objectives: 1) to assure both the uneventful healing of the wound; and 2) the emotional and physical rehabilitation of the patient. The realization of both objectives can be initiated in the immediate postoperative period while the patient is still in the operating room.

RIGID DRESSING

Invariably following surgery, there is considerable swelling in the wound region through extravasation of fluids and the altered hemodynamics. The inflammatory reaction of the healing process adds to this swelling in the later postoperative period. Both problems can be overcome by immediate postoperative application of a rigid dressing. Moreover, the rigid dressing can carry the terminal device, making it into a provisional prosthesis. This is particularly desirable in the upper extremity amputee where prosthetic training, in some instances, can be started on the first postoperative day.

There is a psychological value to the rigid postoperative dressing with a pylon in lower-extremity child amputees. When there is only a soft dressing around the amputation stump, the child is anxious to keep the bed covers up to the hips. It is as if the child is ashamed to let the surrounding people know that part of the limb has been lost. It usually takes some time to induce the child to get out of bed to start walking on crutches.

With a rigid dressing, however, and even though only a pylon is attached to the rigid dressing, the idea of the completeness of the limb seems to be enough to displace the idea of mutilation. Children, in general, are quite willing to show off their newly acquired leg, and are indeed anxious to get out of bed to use it.

The application of the rigid dressing has been well standardized in the literature, and special techniques for various levels of amputation can be learned.[1,2] The principle of the rigid dressing is to cover the sterile dressing over the amputation wound with a sterile absorbent but elastic interface material (reticulated polyurethane or lamb's wool), and then to roll over the remaining part of the limb a sterile orlon lycra stump sock. Bony prominences are protected by establishing reliefs over them, usually by using felt pads. These appliances are covered with a socket of elastic plaster bandages, which are stretched to produce a perfect contour fit. These bandages are reinforced with regular plaster of Paris bandages. The desired fit for the stump is obtained either through manipulation or by the use of casting fixtures.

The suction drain from the amputation wound can be led out of the plaster of Paris socket without trouble, and can be removed without disturbing the cast. If Penrose drains are chosen, it is desirable to remove the drain through a small window in the cast, rather than by removing the cast itself.

The attachment for the terminal device or the terminal device itself can be incorporated into the end of the plaster of Paris socket. In the young and vigorous lower extremity amputee, ambulation with partial weight bearing can be started within 48 hours postoperatively. The patient with circulatory insufficiency, however, should not begin ambulation until after the first change of the rigid dressing, which should take place approximately two weeks after the operation.

The rigid dressing is of value even for a patient two to four weeks after amputation. It decreases the stump edema rapidly and furthers the maturation of the stump. It should be considered in patients who have had secondary closure of an open amputation.

SEMIRIGID DRESSING[3]

When the surgeon is concerned that frequent changes in the postoperative dressing may become necessary, an Unna paste bandage can be used.[3] This bandage is more easily removed, and the reapplication is a less involved and less expensive process than the application of a postoperative rigid dressing. The application of the Unna paste bandage has to be extremely meticulous because no folds in the bandage can be tolerated. The bandage is applied over the wound dressing, and the reliefs for the bony prominences are incorporated in a second layer. The paste is commercially available or can be produced by heating three parts of water and four parts of glycerin together with one part zinc oxide and two parts gelatin in a double boiler. The warm paste has to be spread over each layer of the gauze bandage applied to the remaining part of the limb.

The terminal device cannot be incorporated into the semirigid dressing. If early ambulation is desired in the lower limb amputee, a temporary prosthesis has to be manufactured. It is time-consuming and offsets the cost-saving feature of the Unna paste dressing. Thus, the semirigid dressing may be particularly desirable in those cases where ambulation must be delayed; for example, in the patient with a tenuous blood supply to the stump.

GENERAL CONSIDERATIONS

During the time following the immediate postoperative period, the amputee requires close supervision. The possibility of postoperative hemorrhage is more disastrous the more proximal the amputation. Early signs of circulatory collapse should be looked for constantly. The patient himself should be encouraged to communicate to the staff any unusual signs and symptoms or decrease in his feeling of well-being. At this time, it is advisable to keep an Esmarch bandage at the bedside, and to instruct the nursing staff in the application of the bandage in case of need.

Early ambulation provides a considerable boost to the morale of the patient with a lower extremity amputation. A similar psychological advantage can be derived from the early operation of a terminal device in the upper extremity amputee. Even bed-to-chair activities, however, unipedal crutchwalk, and strengthening exercises for the upper extremities improve the psychological outlook of the patient and his or her energy consumption. Early involvement of the patient in the measurement and manufacturing of the prosthesis has similar advantageous results.

The final steps in the physical rehabilitation of the patient are the fitting, manufacturing, and delivery of the first permanent prosthesis, and the learning of the use of the device.

References

1. Burgess EM, Romano RL, Zettl JH: *Management of lower extremity amputations.* Prosthetic and Surgery Aids Service, Veterans Administration, TR 10-6, 1969.
2. Burgess EM, Romano RL: The management of lower extremity amputees using immediate postsurgical prostheses. *Clin Orthop* 57:137–146, 1968.
3. Ghiulamila RJ: Semi-rigid dressing for postoperative fitting of below-knee prosthesis. *Arch Phys Med Rehab* 53:186–190, 1972.

Part Two
Surgical Techniques

CHAPTER 8
Open Amputation

Open amputations may be necessary when a limb has been severely crushed or grossly contaminated, or when advanced toxicity is present in older people with ischemic limbs. Thus, most war wounds requiring amputation start out as open amputations. It should be a rule to employ open amputation also in farm injuries that are severe enough to require amputation.[1,2]

The aim of the open amputation is to ablate the diseased part of the limb, leaving the amputation wound open and letting it heal either by secondary intention or after a second or third surgical procedure. The open amputation may have to be carried out as a lifesaving procedure, at times with minimal anesthesia, as rapidly as possible. In such cases, a circular open amputation would be applicable.

CIRCULAR OPEN AMPUTATION

The skin incision is carried out approximately 2 cm distally from the intended level of bone transection (Fig. 8-1). The skin is retracted gently; at the level of the retracted skin edge, the musculature is incised down to the bone. The blood vessels are clamped and tied as they are encountered. The bone is then transected (Fig. 8-2). The nerves are dissected free and cut above the level of the amputation. The wound surface is covered with nonadherent gauze, such as Owens gauze or petrolated gauze (Fig. 8-3). Skin adherent is put on the skin of the stump. It is used to hold a stockinette in place. The dressing of the wound is completed with fluffed gauze, and the stockinette is tied over the fluffed gauze. The knot at the end of the stockinette is used to hold in place the cord for skin traction of 1 to 2 kg (Fig. 8-4).

In the postoperative period, care has to be taken to avoid accumulation of wound drainage under the dependent part of the stump. The wound itself is dressed for the first time after two or three days. Skin traction has to be maintained for as long as the wound is in the process of healing. If healing by secondary intention is allowed, the ensuing scar is inverted, unsightly, and usually adherent to the bone. After 10 to 14 days, when granulations appear, revision of the stump can be hastened by placing a meshed skin graft on the end of the stump.

Figures 8-1 to 8-4.   Circular amputation of "Guillotine amputation." The procedure is shown at the below-knee level.

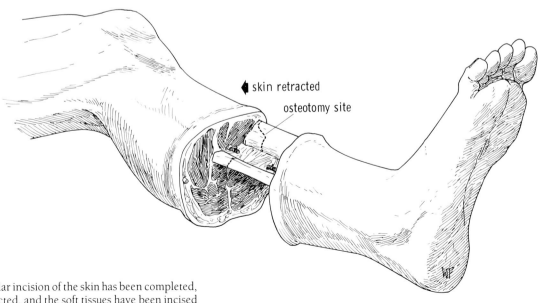

Figure 8-1.   The circular incision of the skin has been completed, the skin has been retracted, and the soft tissues have been incised down to the bone. The level of transection of tibia and fibula as well as the bevel of the tibial crest are indicated.

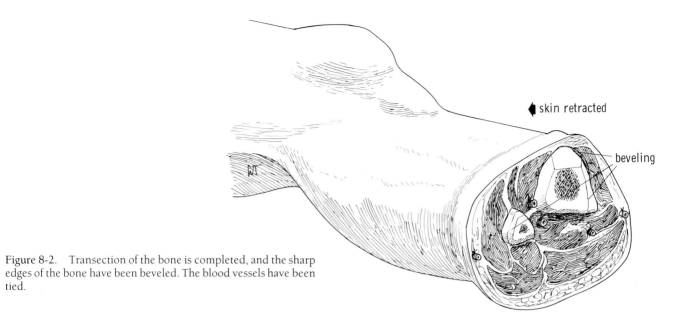

skin retracted

beveling

Figure 8-2.   Transection of the bone is completed, and the sharp edges of the bone have been beveled. The blood vessels have been tied.

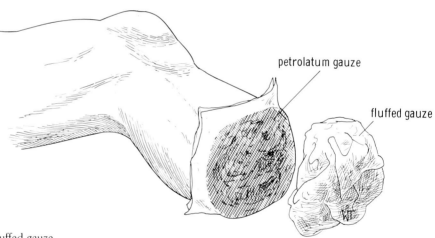

petrolatum gauze

fluffed gauze

Figure 8-3.   Dressing with petrolated and fluffed gauze.

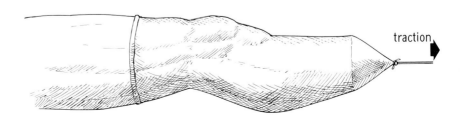

traction

Figure 8-4.   Institution of skin traction.

OPEN FLAP AMPUTATION

In patients with severe crush injuries where there is compromised circulation, the fashioning of standard skin flaps may be impossible. However, the use of atypical skin flaps is preferable to an amputation at a higher level.

The technique of the open flap amputation is somewhat similar to the circular open amputation. Skin flaps are fashioned of sufficient length to cover the amputation wound later on. The underlying soft tissue is transected; and in the process, blood vessels are sought out, clamped, tied, and transected (Fig. 8-5). The nerves are dissected free and transected within the soft tissue above the level of amputation. Where necessary, the bone is transected, and the cut end of the bone is fashioned in such a way that there are no sharp prominences. Five or six No. 1 nonabsorbable sutures are then inserted into the opposing edges of the skin flap, but are not tied (Fig. 8-6).

The wound is covered with Owens or petrolated gauze. Fluffed gauze is placed on top of it, keeping it packed loosely under the skin flaps and the sutures (Fig. 8-7). Skin adherent is placed over the remaining part of the limb, but not the skin flaps themselves. The skin adherent keeps in place a stockinette that serves as an outer dressing as well as a means of skin traction (Fig. 8-8). This traction should be no more than 1 to 2 kg.

There is usually fluid accumulation under the dependent part of the stump. If it is not eliminated, it can lead to maceration of the skin and loosening of the stockinette. After two or three days, the stockinette should be opened and the gauze dressing changed. Care should be taken not to disrupt the skin sutures. The wound should be washed with normal saline, and traction should be resumed after the dressing change.

When healthy granulations appear after 10 to 14 days, and no sign of infection appears, the dressing is removed and the skin flaps are laid over the granulations. The previously inserted No. 1 sutures are gently tied. Frequently, this procedure can eliminate the need of skin closure under anesthesia. It also improves the appearance of the scar.

Figures 8-5 to 8-8.   Open-flap amputation.

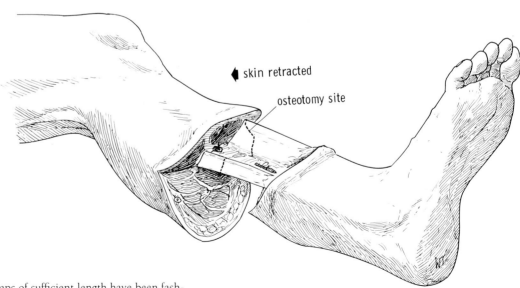

skin retracted

osteotomy site

Figure 8-5.   Soft tissue flaps of sufficient length have been fashioned. The level of transection and the beveling of the tibia are indicated.

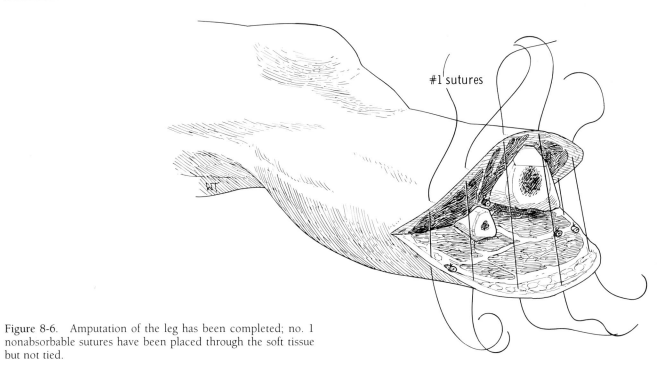

#1 sutures

Figure 8-6. Amputation of the leg has been completed; no. 1 nonabsorbable sutures have been placed through the soft tissue but not tied.

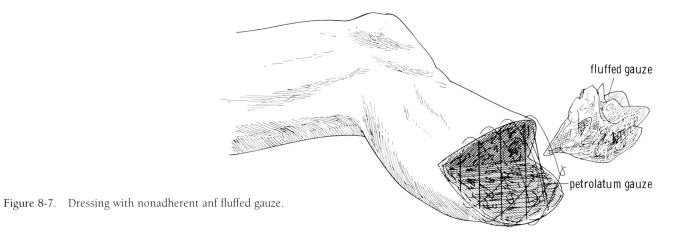

fluffed gauze

petrolatum gauze

Figure 8-7. Dressing with nonadherent anf fluffed gauze.

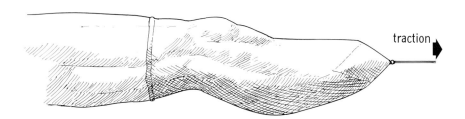

traction

Figure 8-8. Skin traction in place.

OPEN AMPUTATION WITH INVERTED SKIN FLAPS

It has been recommended[3] to invert the skin flaps at the time of surgery by placing interrupted catgut sutures through both the skin edges and the subcutaneous tissue at the base of the skin flap (Fig. 8-9). Dressing of the wound and skin traction is carried out as outlined above. The patient is taken back to the operating room after healthy granulations cover the amputation wound. The catgut sutures are removed, and the inverted skin flaps are unfolded and sutured over the granulation tissue.

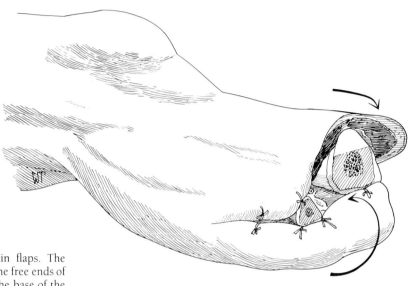

Figure 8-9. Open amputation with inverted skin flaps. The below-knee amputation has been completed, and the free ends of the skin flaps have been inverted and sutured to the base of the flaps.

References

1. Brown PW: Rehabilitation of bilateral lower extremity amputees. *J Bone Joint Surg* 52A:687–700, 1970.
2. Welch RB, Metz CW, Becker QH, Rankin EA: The management of the battle incurred lower extremity amputee. *J Bone Joint Surg* 51A:1041, 1969.
3. Crenshaw AH (ed): Campbells Operative Orthopaedics, 7th ed, vol. 1, C. V. Mosby, 1987, pp 601–603.

CHAPTER 9
Toe Amputation

The general principles of toe amputations are easily explained. Well-vascularized tissue, preferably plantar skin, should be used to cover the amputation stump. The constant pressure of shoes will lead to movement of the neighboring toes into the empty space where the amputated toe was, and varus and valgus deformities of the surrounding toes frequently occur. Thus, it is desirable to preserve parts of the toes, even if they are only used as spacers.

Amputations in the distal or proximal interphalangeal joint may lead to extension contractures of the remaining part of the toes that require tenotomies. This tendency toward dorsal subluxation of the remnant of the toe quickly leads to pressure necroses in patients with vascular insufficiency. Therefore, it is advisable to perform disarticulations in the metatarsophangeal joint in patients with vascular insufficiency, except in the first toe where the proximal phalanx is usually well enough powered and balanced so that it can be maintained.[1]

TECHNIQUE

The joint is opened through a dorsal incision over the joint line. The extensor tendon is transected. Then the collateral ligaments of the joint are transected, and the incision is continued in the midmedial and midlateral line of the toe. A sufficiently large plantar flap is formed to cover the amputation wound. The bone is dissected out of the plantar flap, and the amputation is completed at the distal end of the plantar flap. The flexor tendon is pulled into the wound and transected as far proximally as possible (Fig. 9-1).

It is important to dissect free, and to transect the digital nerves as far proximally as possible. At the same time, the digital arteries and veins can be ligated. The cartilage on the joint surface of the remaining bone is maintained as long as it is glistening and viable, because it decreases the surface of the wound and may act as a barrier against infection for

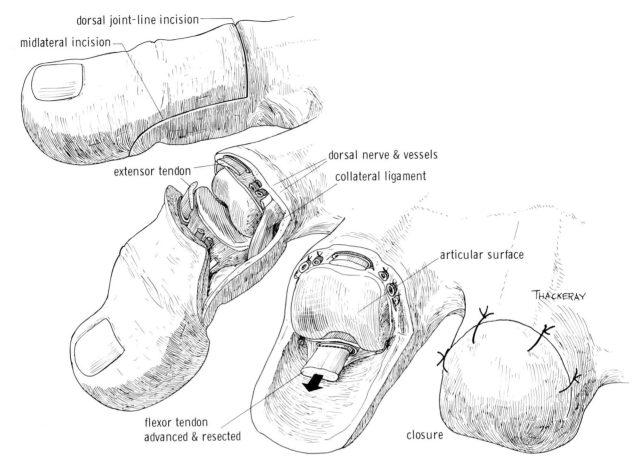

dorsal joint-line incision

midlateral incision

extensor tendon

dorsal nerve & vessels

collateral ligament

articular surface

THACKERAY

flexor tendon
advanced & resected

closure

Figure 9-1.   Four steps in the disarticulation of a toe.

the remaining bone, particularly in patients with vascular insufficiency. The amputation is completed by folding the skin flap from the plantar surface over the exposed part of the bone, and then attaching it to the dorsal skin with a few skin sutures after a small drain has been placed into the wound. This drain should remain in place for approximately 48 hours.

References

1. Baumgartner R: *Beinamputationen und Prothesenversorgung bei arteriellen Durchblutungsstörungen*. Ferdinand Enke, Stuttgart, 1973.

CHAPTER 10
Metatarsal Ray Resection

Resection of part or all of a metatarsal ray can be done in cases of recurrent plantar ulcerations that have led to both a localized osteomyelitis and destruction of the metatarsophalangeal joint. Another indication is the presence of local gigantism. The aim of the surgical procedure is to eradicate the disease by resection within the healthy tissue. At the same time, wound closure must be made possible without causing tension upon the flaps. In the case of an infection, irrigation tubes are placed into the wound.

It is desirable to leave behind enough of the base of the metatarsal bone in order to avoid shifting of the remaining tarsometatarsal joints. Tendons that insert into the first and fifth metatarsal bones will have to be reinserted if the origin has been resected. Patients with ray resections require molded foot orthoses following the operation. This is particularly true for those patients who have had resections on the medial side of the foot.[1,2] However, in dysvascular and insensate feet, resection of the first ray or the first and second rays is usually unsuccessful, because the altered weight bearing leads to skin breakdown and reinfection.

TECHNIQUE

In the case of plantar ulceration, a raquet-type incision must be used. It exposes on the dorsum the amount of metatarsal shaft that needs to be resected. The incision circles the involved toe and includes the ulcer within a sound margin. The metatarsal shaft is exposed as little as possible (Fig. 10-1). The resection should be at least extraperiosteal. When necessary, the intrinsic muscles surrounding the ray are resected en bloc (Fig. 10-2). The metatarsal shaft is transected with an oscillating saw at the desired level (Fig. 10-3), and the ray is resected sharply and bluntly (Fig. 10-4) and lifted out of its bed as a unit (Fig. 10-5). Hemostasis is obtained after release of the tourniquet. Formation of a hematoma, which could become a breeding ground for a new infection in the empty space, must be avoided. The wound is closed over an irrigation system (Fig. 10-6).

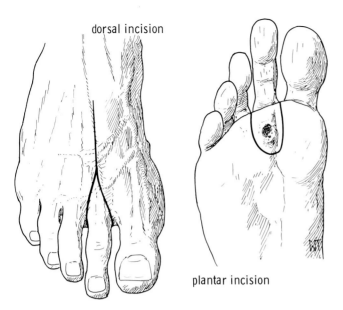

dorsal incision

plantar incision

Figure 10-1. Ray resection in the case of a trophic ulcer under the second metatarsal head. The racquet-shaped incision is shown.

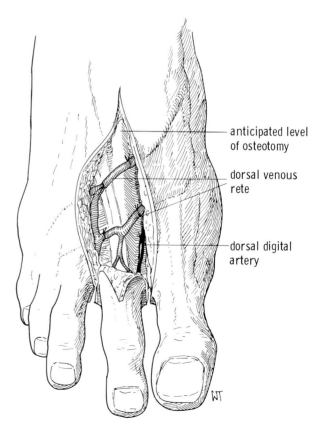

anticipated level of osteotomy

dorsal venous rete

dorsal digital artery

Figure 10-2. The dorsum of the ray is exposed.

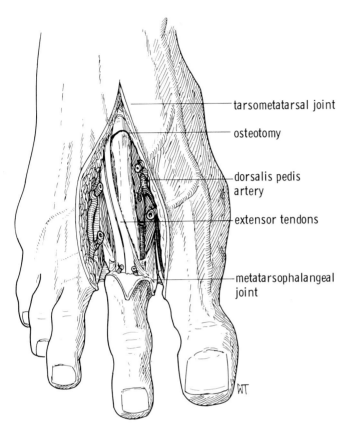

Figure 10-3.   The level of transection of the second metatarsal indicated after the overlaying blood vessels have been cut and tied.

tarsometatarsal joint

osteotomy

dorsalis pedis artery

extensor tendons

metatarsophalangeal joint

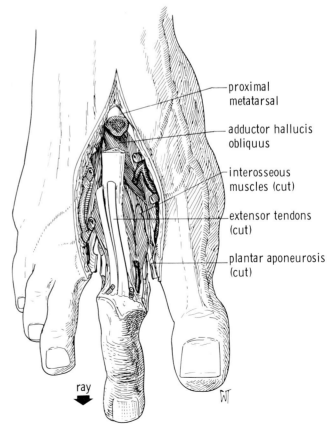

proximal metatarsal

adductor hallucis obliquus

interosseous muscles (cut)

extensor tendons (cut)

plantar aponeurosis (cut)

ray

Figure 10-4.   The intrinsic muscles surrounding the second metatarsal are left attached.

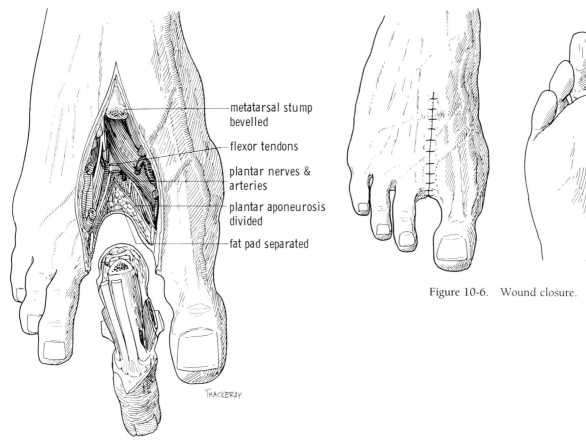

metatarsal stump
bevelled

flexor tendons

plantar nerves &
arteries

plantar aponeurosis
divided

fat pad separated

THACKERAY

Figure 10-5.   The second ray is lifted out of its bed en bloc.

Figure 10-6.   Wound closure.

In the case of local gigantism, the resection is more wedge shaped. The amount of skin resected from the dorsal and plantar side of the foot depends on the extent of the hypertrophy. If no infection is present before the operation, one can decrease the dead space following the wedge resection by osteotomy of the neighboring metatarsals or by sutures through the distal ends of the neighboring metatarsal bones to approximate them.

References

1. Robson MC, Edstrom LE: The diabetic foot: An alternative approach to major amputation. *Surg Clin North Am* 57:1089–1102, 1977.
2. Wagner FW: Amputations of the foot and ankle. *Clin Orthopaedics* 122:62–69, 1977.

CHAPTER 11
Tarsal and Metatarsal Amputations

TRANSMETATARSAL AMPUTATIONS

Transmetatarsal amputations are designed to let the patient walk without a prosthesis. A well-vascularized and sensate stump is necessary. The level of the transmetatarsal amputation is of no great importance as long as the covering plantar flap is of adequate thickness. On the other hand, in the patient with vascular insufficiency, amputation between the proximal and middle one-third of the metatarsal bones promises the best success. The tendons that attach themselves at the base of the first and fifth metatarsal must retain their function. The amputation scar should be on the dorsum of the remaining part of the foot.

Technique[1-3]

The incision crosses the metatarsal bones on the dorsum of the foot at the level of their amputation (Figs. 11-1 and 11-2). It is carried through the tendons down to the bones. Numerous veins on the dorsum of the foot are ligated, as is the dorsalis pedis artery (Figs. 11-3 and 11-4). The metatarsal bones themselves are transected either with a Gigli saw or with an oscillating saw, so that an even line results. The plantar edges of the proximal stumps of the metatarsals are beveled (Fig. 11-5). Both the medial edge in the first metatarsal and the lateral edge in the fifth metatarsal also need to be beveled. The shafts of the metatarsal bones are very brittle, so that the use of bone cutters or chisels usually leads to splintering. The lateral and medial incision of the skin is made somewhat dorsally, and the plantar incision is somewhat distally to the metatarsophalangeal joints. The distal bone ends can now be avulsed out of the wound (Fig. 11-6), and the subcutaneous tissue of the plantar flap can be transected (Fig. 11-7). The neurovascular bundles of the common digital nerves and arteries are identified, the vessels are ligated, and the nerves are resected as far proximally as possible. The flexor tendons are pulled into the wound and transected, and the plantar skin flap is brought over the distal ends of the metatarsals (Fig. 11-8) after a drain has been inserted into either end of the wound. Subcutaneous sutures and skin sutures follow.

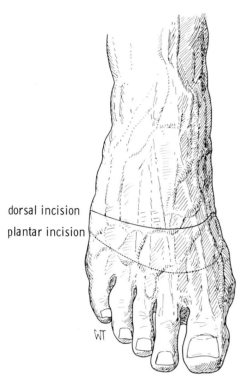

dorsal incision

plantar incision

Figure 11-1.   Placement of the skin incision in relation to the metatarsals.

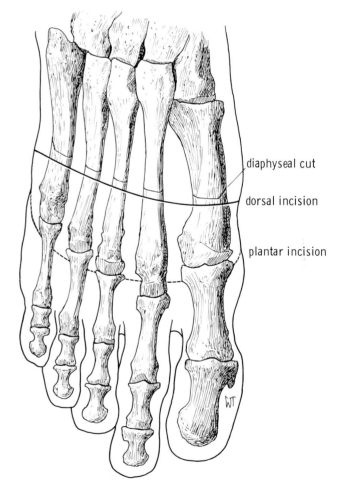

diaphyseal cut

dorsal incision

plantar incision

Figure 11-2.   Placement of the skin incision in relation to the diaphyseal cut.

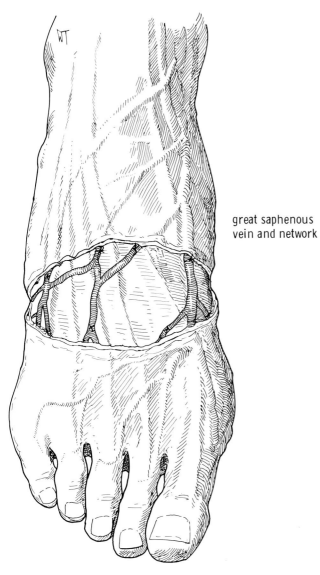

great saphenous
vein and network

Figure 11-3.   The skin is incised and the veins are tied.

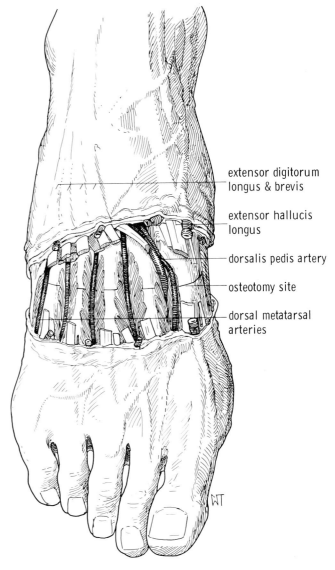

extensor digitorum
longus & brevis

extensor hallucis
longus

dorsalis pedis artery

osteotomy site

dorsal metatarsal
arteries

Figure 11-4.   The soft tissues on the dorsum of the foot have been transected and the veins cut, and the arteries are in view. The level of transection of the metatarsal bones is indicated.

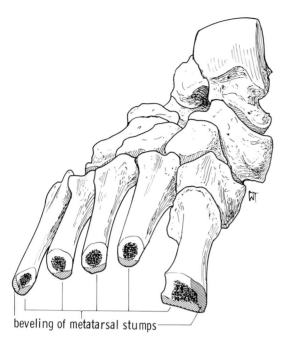

beveling of metatarsal stumps

Figure 11-5.   Beveling of the stumps of the metatarsals.

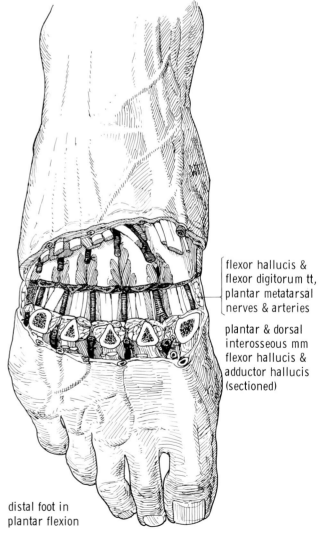

flexor hallucis &
flexor digitorum tt,
plantar metatarsal
nerves & arteries

plantar & dorsal
interosseous mm
flexor hallucis &
adductor hallucis
(sectioned)

distal foot in
plantar flexion

Figure 11-6.   The distal ends of the metatarsals are avulsed out of the wound, and the soft tissue on the plantar surface are transected.

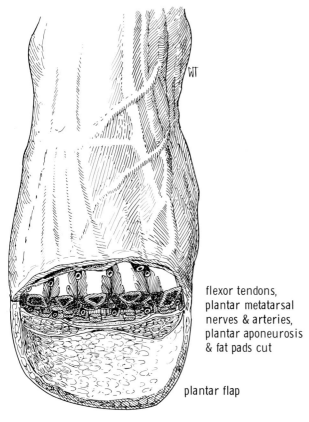

flexor tendons,
plantar metatarsal
nerves & arteries,
plantar aponeurosis
& fat pads cut

plantar flap

Figure 11-7. View of the complete amputation site prior to skin closure.

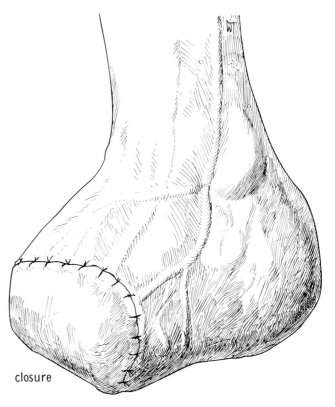

closure

Figure 11-8. Completed skin closure.

THE LISFRANC AND CHOPART AMPUTATIONS

The Lisfranc amputation is carried out through the tarsometatarsal joints. Unless the muscle power of the remaining dorsiflexors is augmented by insertion of the extensor digitorum into the remaining part of the tarsal bones, the stump will assume an equinus position (Fig. 11-9). This position is frequently worsened by a varus deformity, since the medially inserting muscles are insufficiently counterbalanced after the removal of the insertion of the peroneal tendons. Thus, this operation, as well as the Chopart amputation (Fig. 11-10) through the midtarsal joints, is rarely, if ever, indicated.

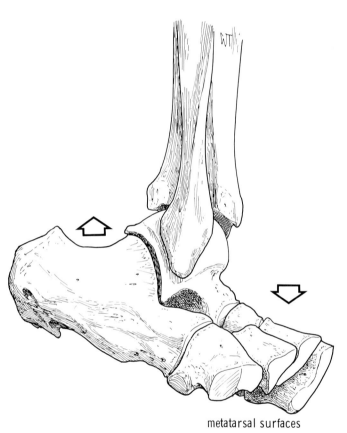

metatarsal surfaces

Figure 11-9.   Lisfranc amputation. Arrows demonstrate the imbalance between the dorsiflexors and plantar flexors of the foot.

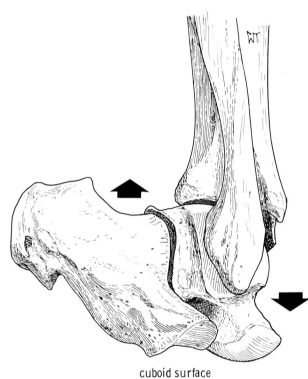

cuboid surface
navicular surface

Figure 11-10.   Chopart amputation. Arrows demonstrate the imbalance between the dorsiflexors and plantar flexors of the foot.

References

1. Effoney DJ, Lim RC, Schecter WP: Transmetatarsal amputation. *Arch Surg* 112:1366–1370, 1977.

2. Wagner FW: Amputations of the foot and ankle. *Clin Orthopaedics* 122:62–69, 1977.

3. Young AE: Transmetatarsal amputation in the management of peripheral ischemia. *Am J Surg* 134:604–607, 1977.

CHAPTER 12
Amputations Around the Ankle

THE PIROGOFF AMPUTATION

The principle of the Pirogoff amputation is the creation of an arthrodesis between the distal end of the tibia and tuber calcanei by rotating the tuber calcanei almost 90°, and allowing it to fuse to the denuded inferior surface of the tibia. As with all amputations that try to preserve the heel pad, extreme care must be taken not to injure the posterior tibial neurovascular bundle (Fig. 12-1). This provides the main lifeline to the heel pad after the operation.

An advantage of the surgical procedure is that there is little, if any, decrease of the overall length of the leg. However, since the posterior aspect of the heel is ultimately used for weight bearing, the true heel pad is no longer in the weight-bearing line.

Technique

From the tip of the lateral malleolus, the incision passes over the anterior aspect of the ankle joint, and then medially to a point 1 cm below the medial malleolus. This point is then connected with the tip of the lateral malleolus by an incision through the plantar skin in the coronal plane. The incision is carried to the bone (Fig. 12-2).

The medial and lateral collateral ligaments are severed by inserting the blade of the knife between the talus and the medial and lateral malleolus, respectively (Fig. 12-3). Care must be taken not to push the knife blade too far posteriorly on the medial side, since the neurovascular bundle is in the immediate vicinity of the medial malleolus. After transection of the ligament, the foot can be plantarflexed strongly, and the posterior part of the capsule of the ankle joint comes into view. This is opened, and the superior surface of the tuber calcanei comes into view (Fig. 12-4).

Approximately one-third to one-half of the tuber calcanei is stripped of its periosteum, narrow Bennett retractors are inserted subperiosteally, and the tuber calcanei is transected sharply with an osteotome (Fig. 12-5). The foot can now be removed, excluding the posterior part of the tuber calcanei.

The ankle mortise is now exposed subperiosteally. Care must be taken not to injure the posterior tibial neurovascular bundle in the process. The tibia and fibula are transected approximately 2 cm above the tibial plafond. The posterior tibial vessels are ligated in the wound; the posterior tibial nerve is dissected free and cut away from the suture line. Similarly, the veins of the dorsum of the foot are ligated, and the branches of the peroneal nerve and sural and saphenous nerves are cut back. The tourniquet is released, and further hemostasis is obtained. The cut surface of the tuber calcanei is approximated to the cut surface of the tibia and held in place either by interrupted sutures through the periosteum of both structures or by a Steinmann pin reaching through the tuber calcanei into the marrow cavity of the tibia (Fig. 12-6). The suction drain is introduced into the wound through a posterolateral stab wound. The wound is closed with interrupted absorbable, subcutaneous, and nonabsorbable skin sutures (Fig. 12-7).

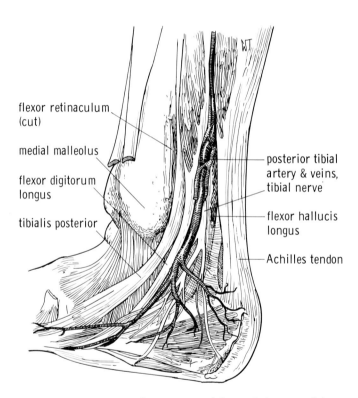

flexor retinaculum
(cut)

medial malleolus

flexor digitorum
longus

tibialis posterior

posterior tibial
artery & veins,
tibial nerve

flexor hallucis
longus

Achilles tendon

Figure 12-1.   Topographic anatomy of the medial aspect of the ankle. Note the juxtaposition of the posterior tibial artery to the deltoid ligament.

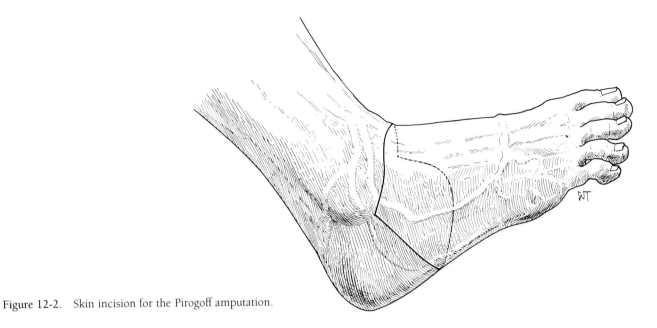

Figure 12-2. Skin incision for the Pirogoff amputation.

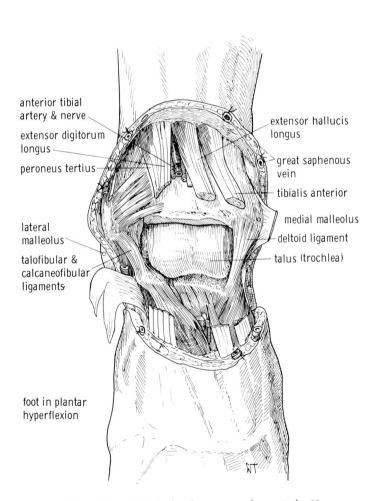

anterior tibial
artery & nerve

extensor digitorum
longus

peroneus tertius

lateral
malleolus

talofibular &
calcaneofibular
ligaments

foot in plantar
hyperflexion

extensor hallucis
longus

great saphenous
vein

tibialis anterior

medial malleolus

deltoid ligament

talus (trochlea)

Figure 12-3. The ankle joint has been opened anteriorly. Note
the medial and lateral collateral ligaments.

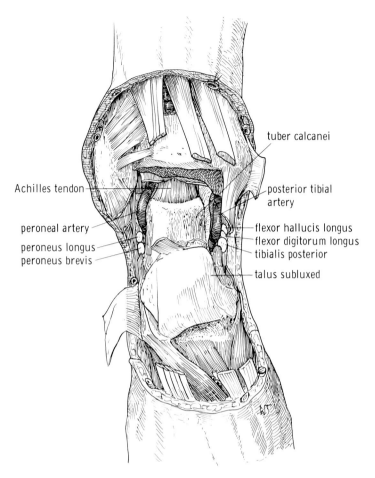

Figure 12-4.   The top of the tubercalcanei is exposed.

tuber calcanei

Achilles tendon

posterior tibial artery

peroneal artery

peroneus longus
peroneus brevis

flexor hallucis longus
flexor digitorum longus
tibialis posterior

talus subluxed

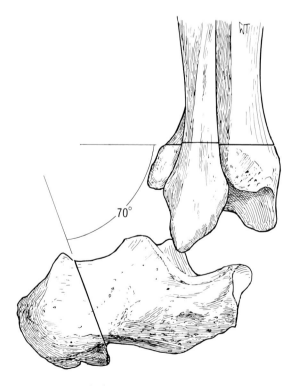

70°

Figure 12-5.   Level of transection of the ankle mortise and the tubercalcanei.

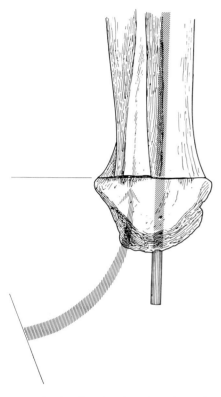

Figure 12-6.   The distal end of the tubercalcanei has been fitted under the tibia and is held in place by a Steinmann pin.

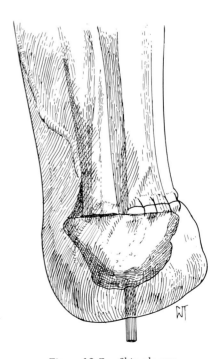

Figure 12-7.   Skin closure.

THE BOYD AMPUTATION

In an attempt to overcome the disadvantage of the Pirogoff amputation, which uses the posterior rather than the plantar aspect of the heel as a weight-bearing surface, Boyd recommended excision of the talus together with the rest of the foot.[1,2] However, the greater part of the calcaneus should be fused to the ankle mortise in its anatomic orientation. This greatly improves the weight-bearing characteristics of the heel pad. This procedure is applicable to the child as well as to the adult. In the adult, the fitting of a prosthesis is rather difficult, and the patient usually uses a high-top shoe with a cosmetic filler. The child with the Boyd amputation and a severely shortened extremity does very well with a prosthesis.

Originally, Boyd recommended talectomy through a Kocher incision. An easier approach, however, appears to be a talectomy through the dorsal part of the incision for removal of the foot.

Technique

The incision starts anteriorly from the tip of the lateral malleolus, proceeds over the dorsum of the foot at the level of the talonavicular joint, and continues medially to the anterior aspect of the medial malleolus. The plantar part of the incision continues from the end of the dorsal incision at the medial malleolus, around the plantar aspect of the foot at the level of the tarsometatarsal joint to end at the lateral malleolus (Fig. 12-8). The incision is carried through the soft tissue to the bone. The dorsal soft tissue flap is raised to approach the ankle joint and to open the anterior part of its capsule (Fig. 12-9). The talus is mobilized by inserting the knife blade between the talus and the malleoli, and then transecting the ligaments on the medial and lateral side. Care has to be taken to preserve the posterior tibial neurovascular bundle. The ankle can now be subluxated out of the mortise, and the posterior part of the capsule can be transected (Fig. 12-10). The talus and calcaneus can now be separated slightly, and the scalpel can be inserted between the talus and calcaneus to transect the talocalcaneal ligament. Thereafter, the talus can easily be removed with the rest of the foot (Fig. 12-11).

A 1 to 1.5 cm thick slice must be removed from the anterior part of the calcaneus. A burr is used to denude the ankle mortise and the superior surface of the calcaneus from all cartilage (Fig. 12-12). The sustentaculum tali may need to be trimmed to fit the top of the calcaneus into the ankle mortise. The calcaneus must be pulled forward to fit into the mortise.

The tendons are drawn into the wound, transected, and allowed to retract. The dorsalis pedis artery, the veins of the dorsum of the foot, and the posterior tibial vessels are ligated. The posterior tibial nerve, as well as the cutaneous nerves in the dorsal flap, are dissected free and cut back. The tourniquet is removed and hemostasis is obtained.

The calcaneus is now fitted into the ankle mortise. It is held in place by a heavy Kirschner wire from the plantar aspect into the medullary cavity of the tibia (Fig. 12-13). The wound is closed using interrupted absorbable sutures for the subcutaneous tissue and nonabsorbable sutures for the skin (Fig. 12-14).

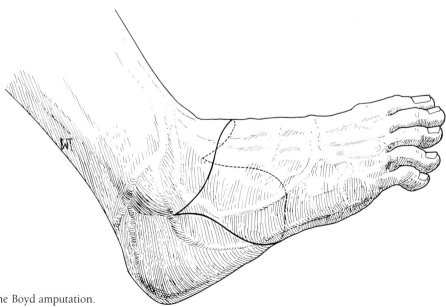

Figure 12-8.   Skin incision for the Boyd amputation.

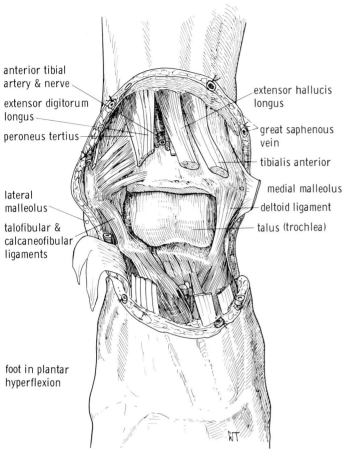

anterior tibial
artery & nerve

extensor digitorum
longus

peroneus tertius

lateral
malleolus

talofibular &
calcaneofibular
ligaments

foot in plantar
hyperflexion

extensor hallucis
longus

great saphenous
vein

tibialis anterior

medial malleolus

deltoid ligament

talus (trochlea)

Figure 12-9. The capsule of the ankle joint has been opened anteriorly.

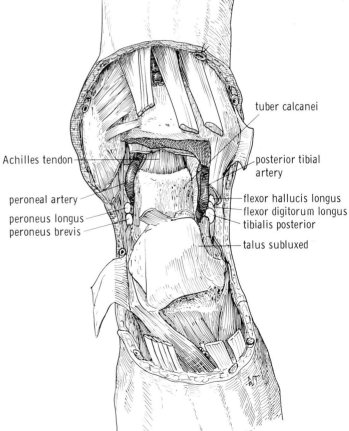

Achilles tendon

peroneal artery

peroneus longus
peroneus brevis

tuber calcanei

posterior tibial
artery

flexor hallucis longus
flexor digitorum longus
tibialis posterior

talus subluxed

Figure 12-10. The collateral ligaments have been transected; the posterior capsule has been opened.

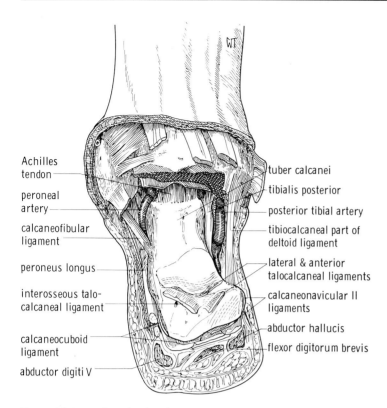

Achilles
tendon

peroneal
artery

calcaneofibular
ligament

peroneus longus

interosseous talo-
calcaneal ligament

calcaneocuboid
ligament

abductor digiti V

tuber calcanei

tibialis posterior

posterior tibial artery

tibiocalcaneal part of
deltoid ligament

lateral & anterior
talocalcaneal ligaments

calcaneonavicular II
ligaments

abductor hallucis

flexor digitorum brevis

Figure 12-11.   The talus has been removed with the rest of the foot. The
calcaneus remains.

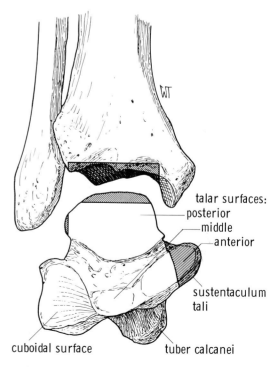

talar surfaces:
posterior
middle
anterior

sustentaculum
tali

cuboidal surface

tuber calcanei

Figure 12-12.   The shaded areas are to be resected.

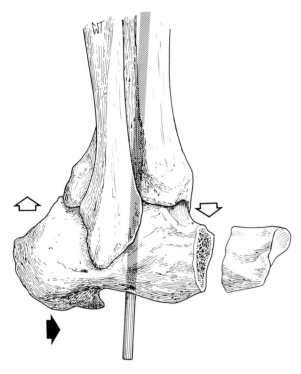

Figure 12-13. The tubercalcanei has been pushed forward into the ankle mortise and fixed with a Steinmann pin. The anterior process of the calcaneus has been resected.

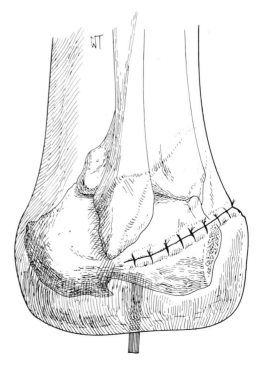

Figure 12-14.   Skin closure.

THE SYME AMPUTATION

The Syme amputation provides an end-bearing stump at the most proximal level below the knee. The aim of the operation is to remove the entire foot, but preserve the plantar skin of the heel to cover the distal end of the tibia and fibula. It is important to maintain as much of the cancellous bone at the distal end of the tibia and fibula as possible, and to make the cut through the bones parallel to the floor. The disadvantage is that this creates a rather bulbous stump end, and it requires a versatile prosthetist to create the artificial limb. The limb itself is often unsightly. This disadvantage is counterbalanced by the fact that the patient can walk without a prosthesis a fair distance and, even with the prosthesis, has excellent proprioception. Wherever possible, the Syme amputation should be carried out in elderly patients.

To slim down the bulbous stump end, resection of the flair above the ankle mortise has been recommended.[3] This procedure somewhat decreases the weight-bearing surface at the distal end of the stump, increases the ease of prosthetic fitting, and still maintains the proprioceptive properties of the heel pad.

Finally, the concept of the Syme amputation is particularly valuable in children. Disarticulation of the ankle and maintenance of the distal tibial and fibular epiphyses are vastly preferable to a standard below-knee amputation, with its typical problems of overgrowth and spindling of the distal skeletal stump end.[4-7]

Technique

The skin incision starts in front of the lateral malleolus, and continues across the anterior part of the ankle joint to the anterior portion of the medial malleolus. It continues in a vertical line downward through the plantar skin covering the calcaneus (Fig. 12-15). The size of the plantar flap can be varied if sufficient skin is available on the plantar aspect, and if a more extensive area needs to be covered on the dorsal aspect of the ankle. On the plantar aspect, the incision is carried down to the bone. On the dorsal aspect, the tendons of the anterior tibial muscle and extensor digitorum longus are identified and marked with sutures before transection distally to those sutures (Fig. 12-16). The incision is then carried to the bone as well. The ankle joint is opened anteriorly (Fig. 12-17). The lateral ligaments of the ankle are transected by inserting a knife between the talus and lateral malleolus and cutting downward, while keeping the knife close to the talus. The medial ligaments are severed in a similar fashion, although care has to be taken not to injure the posterior tibial artery or veins. After transection of the liagments. the talus can be subluxated downward in the ankle mortise, and the posterior part of the capsule can be incised. Again, it is important to maintain the integrity of the posterior tibial vessels.

Now the tuber calcanei comes into view, and its periosteum is incised and stripped (Fig. 12-18). The Achilles tendon can be seen in the depth, and it should be severed from the tuber calcanei. By sharp

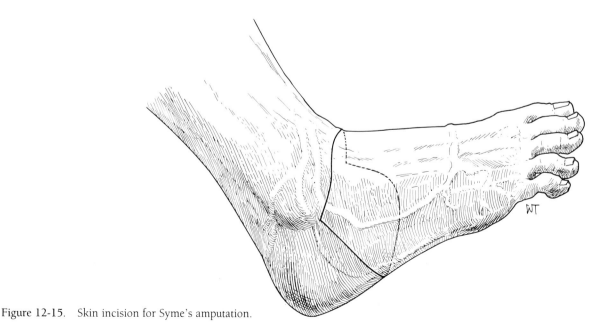

Figure 12-15.   Skin incision for Syme's amputation.

and blunt dissection, the tuber calcanei is fully freed from the plantar skin. With this maneuver, the amputation of the foot is completed (Fig. 12-19).

The posterior tibial tendon, the long flexor tendons on the plantar aspect of the foot, and the peroneal tendons are identified, pulled into the wound, and transected so they can retract into their tendon sheaths. The posterior tibial nerve is dissected free and cut back far enough so as not to be caught in the suture line. The posterior tibial artery, as well as the veins, are ligated (Fig. 12-20). Similarly, the dorsalis pedis artery and the veins in the dorsum of the foot are ligated. The sural nerve and branches of the peroneal nerve on the dorsum of the foot are dissected free and cut back. With a reciprocating saw, the medial and lateral malleolus are removed, together with a thin piece of the joint surface from the distal end of the tibia. The surface of the cut should be at

90° to the line of weight bearing of the lower extremity (Fig. 12-21). The tourniquet is released, and further hemostasis is obtained.

Closure of the wound is started by suturing the stumps of the tendons of both the anterior tibial muscle and the extensor digitorum longus into the periosteum of the plantar surface of the calcaneus (Fig. 12-22). This gives added insurance against a posterior displacement of the heel pad through the pull of the calf musculature. A suction drain is inserted into the dead space between the distal end of the skeletal stump and the heel pad. Interrupted subcutaneous sutures are particularly necessary in this amputation because of the disparity between the thick plantar skin and the much thinner dorsal skin. Interrupted skin sutures complete the wound closure (Fig. 12-23). Wound tapes and plaster of Paris are used to prevent the heel pad from dislocating posteriorly.

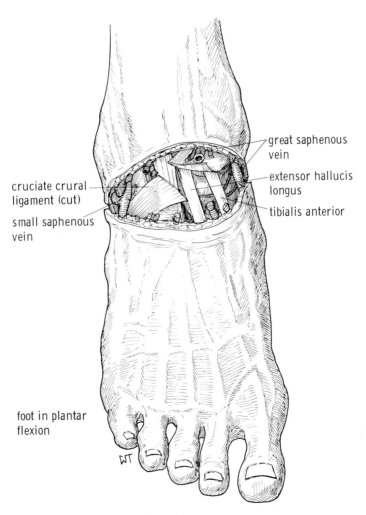

great saphenous vein

extensor hallucis longus

tibialis anterior

cruciate crural ligament (cut)

small saphenous vein

foot in plantar flexion

Figure 12-16. Exposure of the extensor tendons.

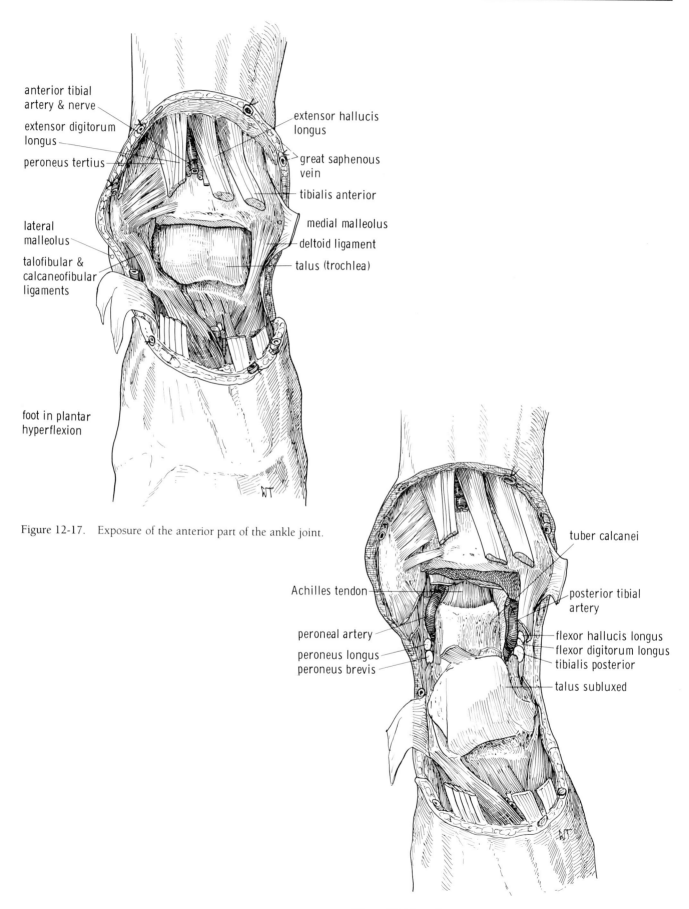

anterior tibial
artery & nerve

extensor digitorum
longus

peroneus tertius

lateral
malleolus

talofibular &
calcaneofibular
ligaments

foot in plantar
hyperflexion

extensor hallucis
longus

great saphenous
vein

tibialis anterior

medial malleolus

deltoid ligament

talus (trochlea)

Figure 12-17.   Exposure of the anterior part of the ankle joint.

Achilles tendon

peroneal artery

peroneus longus
peroneus brevis

tuber calcanei

posterior tibial
artery

flexor hallucis longus
flexor digitorum longus
tibialis posterior

talus subluxed

Figure 12-18.   The ankle joint has been dislocated.

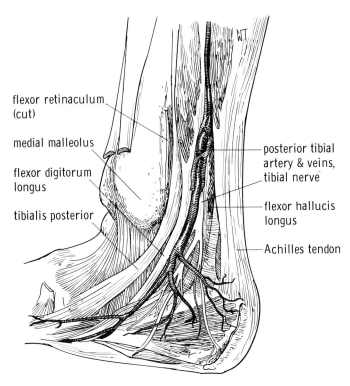

flexor retinaculum (cut)

medial malleolus

flexor digitorum longus

tibialis posterior

posterior tibial artery & veins, tibial nerve

flexor hallucis longus

Achilles tendon

Figure 12-19.   Anatomy around the medial malleolus.

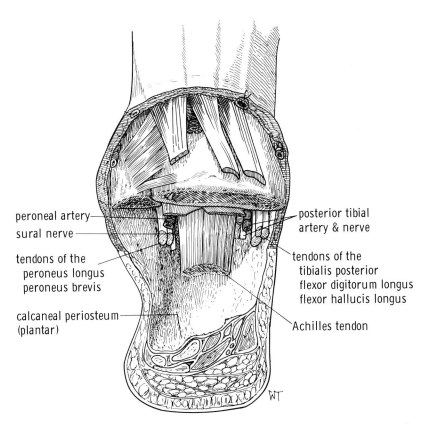

peroneal artery

sural nerve

tendons of the peroneus longus peroneus brevis

calcaneal periosteum (plantar)

posterior tibial artery & nerve

tendons of the tibialis posterior flexor digitorum longus flexor hallucis longus

Achilles tendon

Figure 12-20.   The foot has been removed, and the malleoli have been sawed off.

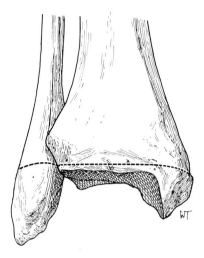

Figure 12-21.   Level of transection at the distal end of the tibia and fibula.

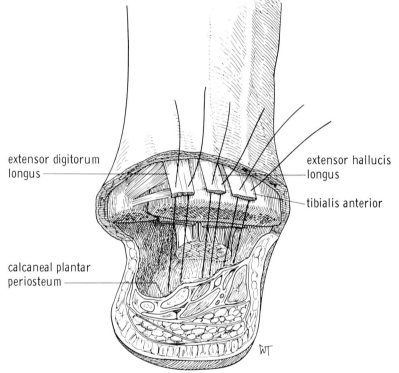

extensor digitorum longus

extensor hallucis longus

tibialis anterior

calcaneal plantar periosteum

Figure 12-22.   The extensor tendons are sewn into the heel pad.

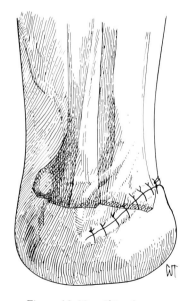

Figure 12-23.   Skin closure.

TWO-STAGE SYME AMPUTATION

Use of the Syme amputation in two stages for the infected dysvascular foot was recommended by Wagner.[3] He outlined eight prerequisites for the procedure to be successful:

1. The patient must be a potential prosthesis user.
2. The heel pad must be free from open lesions.
3. Doppler systolic pressure at the ankle must be at least 70 mm Hg.
4. The ratio of ankle Doppler systolic pressure to the arm systolic pressure must be over 0.45.
5. There should be no gross pus at the amputation site.
6. There should be no ascending lymphangitis.
7. There should be no gas in the tissues above the amputation site by palpation or X-ray examination.
8. Intraoperative bleeding should occur in the skin of the flap within three minutes after release of the tourniquet.

Technique

The first stage of the Syme amputation for the dysvascular foot follows closely that described in the one-step procedure for the treatment of the distal end of the tibia and fibula. These are left intact. If the protruding malleoli cause displacement of the heel flap, Wagner recommends straight incisions into the fat pad to allow nesting of the malleoli. An inflow drain is placed into the wound cavity through a posterolateral incision above the ankle joint. An outflow drain through the wound is left to evacuate the inflowing antiobiotic solution through gravity. No attempt is made to trim the corners of the skin at the suture line.

The second stage takes place after six weeks, and after solid wound healing has occurred. Medial and lateral incisions are made over the protruding corners of the skin and carried down to the malleoli. The malleoli are outlined sharply and then removed flush with the ankle joint. The flare above each one of the malleoli is removed with an osteotome and a rongeur. This squares the distal end of the skeletal stump. If the heel pad is unstable, it can be sutured to the bone through drill holes. The skin edges are excised, and the skin is closed with interrupted nonabsorbable sutures. A walking cast is applied after 7 to 10 days.

SYME AMPUTATION IN CHILDREN

In the child with a congenital deformity of the lower extremity, a modified Syme amputation may be indicated. This procedure aims at disarticulation of the talus from the ankle mortise, but still maintains the heel flap as the weight-bearing area. Thus, the distal tibial and, if present, fibular epiphyses are maintained, and the bone continues to grow commensurately with the soft tissues. The procedure follows closely that described for the adult.[8,9]

The skin incision may need to be modified in cases of congenital absence of the fibula, where the bony landmark of the lateral malleolus is missing. The incision should lie in a coronal plane through the anterior margin of the ankle.

After opening the ankle joint and transection of the medial and lateral collateral ligaments of the ankle, the calcaneus is again removed subperiosteally. If desired, the apophysis of the calcaneus can be preserved and drawn with the heel pad under the ankle. No attempt should be made to resect the malleoli or any part of the distal end of the tibia to avoid injury to the distal epiphyses.

In children, it appears particularly important to provide active extension of the heel pad by inserting the anterior tibial tendon and the toe extensor tendons into the heel pad to counterbalance the pull of the triceps surae. Wound closure and drainage should be carried out as previously described for the adult.

References

1. Boyd HB: Amputations of the foot, with calcaneotibial arthrodesis. *J Bone Joint Surg* 21:977–1000, 1939.
2. Eilert RE, Jayakumar SS: Boyd and Syme ankle amputations in children. *J Bone Joint Surg* 58-A:1138–1141, 1976.
3. Wagner FW: Amputations of the foot and ankle. *Clin Orthopaedics* 122:62–69, 1977.
4. Syme J: Amputation at the ankle joint. *London Edinburgh Monthly Med Sci* 3:93–96, 1843.
5. Alldredge RH, Thompson TC: The technique of the Syme amputation. *J Bone Joint Surg* 28:415–426, 1946.
6. Harris RI: Syme's amputation. The technique essential to secure a satisfactory end-bearing stump: Part I. *Can J Surg* 6:456–469, 1963.
7. Harris RI: Syme's amputation. The technique essential to secure a satisfactory end-bearing stump: Part II. *Can J Surg* 7:53–63, 1964.
8. Davidson WH, Bohne WHO: The Syme amputation in children. *J Bone Joint Surg* 57-A:905–909, 1975.
9. Mazet R: Syme's amputation: A follow-up study of fifty-one adults and thirty-two children. *J Bone Joint Surg* 50-A:1549–1563, 1968.

CHAPTER 13
Below the Knee Amputation

The aim of the below-knee amputation is both eradication of the disease process in the distal part of the leg and preservation of an optimally functioning stump. The optimal stump retains approximately 15 to 18 cm of the proximal end of the tibia, is cylindrical or slightly conical in shape, and provides a firm, well-muscled soft tissue mantle with adequate soft tissue coverage at the distal end of the bony stump. The standard procedure will be described for both the limb with adequate circulation as well as the ischemic limb.

NONISCHEMIC LIMBS

With the patient in supine position, a pneumatic tourniquet is applied, and the extremity is suitably prepared and draped. After elevation of the leg, the tourniquet is inflated. The level of the section of the bone is marked at the midlateral and midmedial lines of the lower leg; from there, anterior and posterior flaps of equal length are outlined (Fig. 13-1). It may be advisable to make the flaps longer than preoperatively calculated to ensure their fit. The anterior incision is carried through the subcutaneous tissue, the periosteum over the anteromedial surface of the tibia, and the fascia of the anterior compartment (Fig. 13-2). Skin, periosteum, and fascia are raised as a single layer (Fig. 13-3). The muscles of the anterior compartment are elevated from the undersurface and beveled up to 5 cm distal to the level of the bone section. At this point, the anterior tibial vessels are in view and can be ligated proximally to the level of the bone section. The superficial and deep branch of the peroneal nerve should be dissected free to a level well proximal to the level of the bone section, and then ligated and cut. Next, the tibia is cut at the predetermined level; the fibula is cut 1 to 1.5 cm more proximally (Fig. 13-4). Thereafter, the muscles of the posterior compartment are transected, leaving gastrocnemius and soleus as the longest. Anteriorly to the soleus, the posterior tibial artery and peroneal artery, as well as their associated veins, are found and ligated. Between the two of them, the tibial nerve is dissected free well above the level of the bone section, and then ligated and cut. The saphenous and sural nerves are also found, dissected free, and cut back (Fig. 13-5). At the distal end of the bony stump, the anterior crest of the tibia is now beveled at a 45° angle, and all sharp edges are rounded off. The tourniquet is released and all bleeding points are coagulated.[1]

Tension myodesis is carried out by drilling four or five holes into the distal end of the tibia. Nonabsorbable sutures are passed through these drill holes (Fig. 13-6). The deep portion of the anterior and posterior compartment muscles are fixated with those sutures after these muscles have been put under tension. The gastrocnemius and soleus are then beveled in such a fashion that they can be brought forward and sutured to the fascia of the anterior compartment and to the periosteum of the tibia (Fig. 13-7). A suction drainage tube is placed under the gastrosoleus muscle flap, and is brought out laterally through the skin. Excess skin is excised. However, enough should be left to allow closure without tension. Interrupted sutures are used. A rigid postoperative dressing is applied.

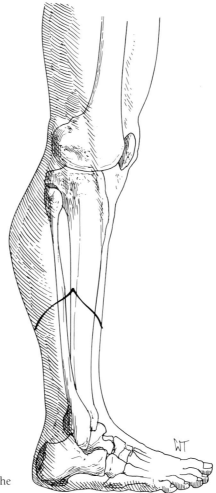

Figure 13-1. Incision for the below-knee amputation in the nonischemic limb.

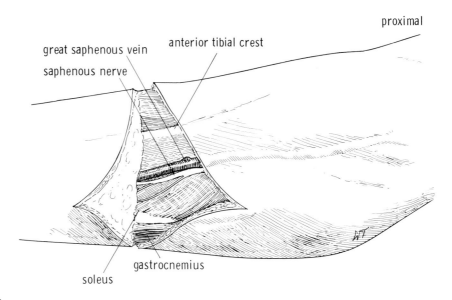

Figure 13-2. Exposure of the subcutaneous structures of the medial side.

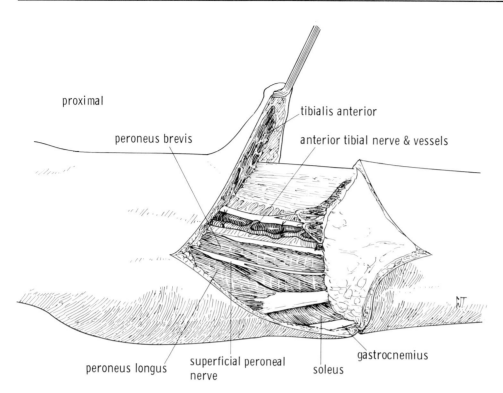

proximal

tibialis anterior

peroneus brevis

anterior tibial nerve & vessels

peroneus longus

superficial peroneal
nerve

soleus

gastrocnemius

Figure 13-3.   Exposure of the subcutaneous tissue on the lateral side. The muscles of the anterior
compartment have been elevated.

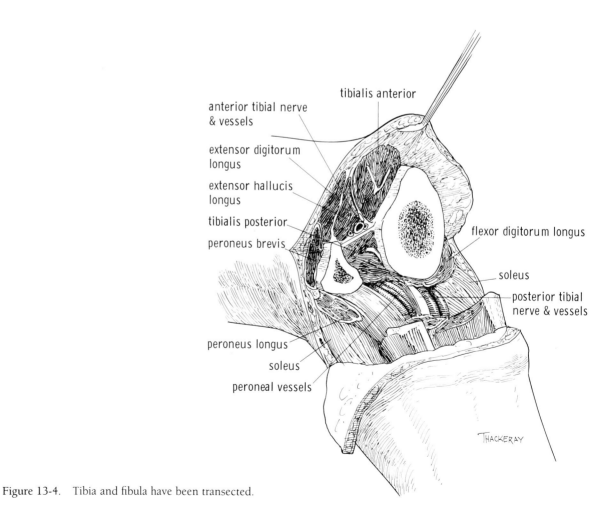

tibialis anterior

anterior tibial nerve
& vessels

extensor digitorum
longus

extensor hallucis
longus

tibialis posterior

peroneus brevis

flexor digitorum longus

soleus

posterior tibial
nerve & vessels

peroneus longus

soleus

peroneal vessels

Figure 13-4.   Tibia and fibula have been transected.

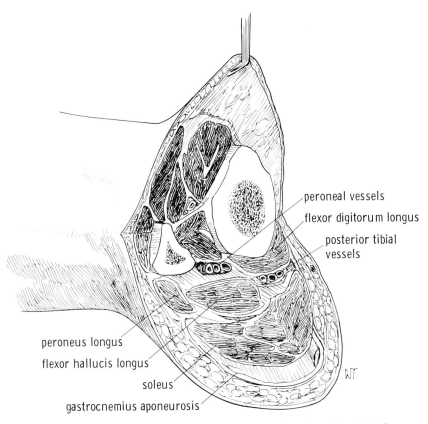

peroneal vessels

flexor digitorum longus

posterior tibial
vessels

peroneus longus

flexor hallucis longus

soleus

gastrocnemius aponeurosis

Figure 13-5. The muscles of the posterior compartment have been beveled. The neurovascular structures of the posterior compartment are ligated.

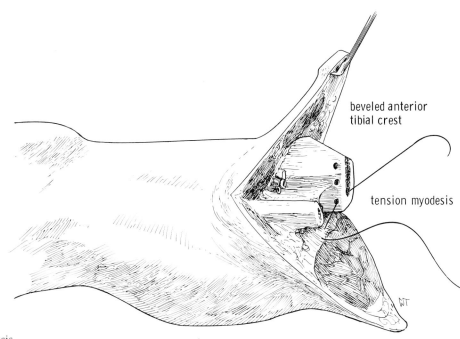

beveled anterior
tibial crest

tension myodesis

Figure 13-6. Myodesis.

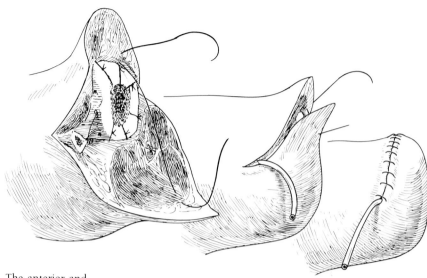

Figure 13-7. Myodesis has been completed. The anterior and posterior rim of the fascia are being sutured together.

ISCHEMIC LIMBS

The goal of amputation in patients with ischemic limbs, of course, is to obtain viable soft tissue flaps that allow primary healing. The best circulation is most likely to be found in the posterior compartment. Therefore, a long posterior flap is recommended. However, lateral flaps of equal length have been recommended, and successful amputations below the knee have been carried out under these circumstances. Indeed, flaps fashioned in an unorthodox manner can be used wherever viable tissue is found to cover the stump end at the time of surgery (Fig. 13-8).[2,3]

Technique

Amputation in the Coronal Plane

With the patient in supine position, a tourniquet is applied around the thigh, but not inflated. The extremity is prepared and draped in a suitable manner. The level of the bony section is marked at approximately 13 to 15 cm distal to the knee joint line. The midmedial and midlateral line of the lower leg is marked at the same point, and the two points are connected over the anterior aspect of the leg. The apex of the posterior flap is approximately 15 cm distal to that line (Fig. 13-9).

The anterior incision divides the skin, subcutaneous tissue, fascia of the anterior compartment, and periosteum over the anteromedial aspect of the tibia in one flap. The anterior compartment muscles are elevated from the interosseous membrane, and the anterior tibial vessels are ligated proximal to the level of bony transection (Fig. 13-3). The superficial and deep branches of the peroneal nerve are dissected free and cut well proximal to the area of bony transection after ligation. Thereafter, the tibia is transected. The fibula is transected approximately 1 to 1.5 cm more proximally (Fig. 13-4). A flap is formed out of the muscles in the posterior aspect of the leg, and the soft tissue is transected, creating the posterior flap. The posterior tibial and peroneal arteries are ligated, and the tibial nerve is tied and cut well proximal of the area of bony transection (Fig. 13-5). The sural nerve and saphenous nerve are dissected free and cut back as well. The anterior tibial crest is beveled at an angle approximately 45°, and all sharp edges are rounded. Hemostasis is obtained, and the posterior compartment muscles are beveled to allow for coverage of the stump end. A suction drainage tube is introduced into the wound under the posterior flap, and is brought out through a separate opening in the skin. The posterior flap is brought forward and sutured anteriorly to both the periosteum of the tibia and fascia of the anterior compartment muscles (Fig. 13-7). The skin should be closed with minimal tension, and excess skin in the midmedial and midlateral lines of the incision should be left intact. The skin is closed with interrupted nonabsorbable sutures. A sterile dressing is applied, and over that a rigid dressing is placed.

Technique

Amputation in the Sagittal Plane[4,5]

With the patient supine and adequately anesthetized, a tourniquet is employed around the thigh, but not inflated. The extremity is prepared and draped in a suitable fashion. The midline of the leg is determined anteriorly and posteriorly. Anteriorly, the midline is approximately 1 cm lateral to the tibial crest. A point approximately 15 cm distally to the knee joint line is marked anteriorly and posteriorly. This is the level of the base of the medial and lateral soft tissue flaps, as well as the level of transection of the tibia. From this level, a point approximately 8 cm distally is marked on the midmedial and midlateral lines of the leg. These points represent the apices of the medial and lateral flap (Fig. 13-10).

The incision is started by cutting the skin, subcutaneous tissue, and fascia cruris perpendicularly. The muscles are cut in such a fashion that they are beveled toward the apices. The medial and lateral flaps can thus be elevated easily, exposing the tibia for transection. The anterior crest of the tibia is beveled at a 45° angle, and the fibula is cut approximately 1 cm further proximally than the tibia. In the anterior compartment, anterior tibial vessels are ligated. The peroneal nerves are transected well above the level of bony transection after they have been ligated. In the posterior compartment, the posterior tibial artery and peroneal artery, as well as tibial nerve, are treated in the same fashion (Fig. 13-11). Hemostasis is obtained. The bone ends are smoothed, and a suction drainage tube is put into the V-shaped wound and brought out through the lateral aspect of the remaining stump. The fascia cruris on the medial and lateral side is approximated with interrupted absorbable sutures, and the skin is closed with nonabsorbable sutures in interrupted fashion. Sterile dressings and a rigid postoperative dressing are applied.

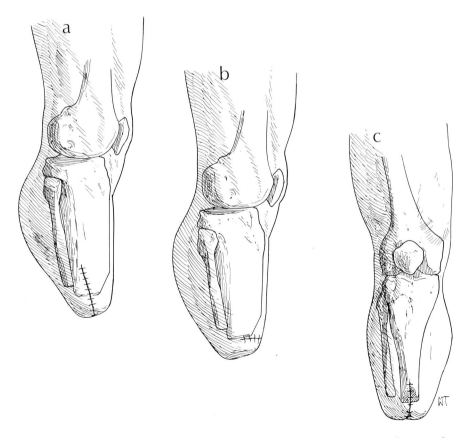

Figure 13-8.   Suture line in the various types of below-knee amputation: a. In the nonischemic limb. b. Amputation of the ischemic limb in the coronal plane. c. Amputation of the ischemic limb in the sagittal plane.

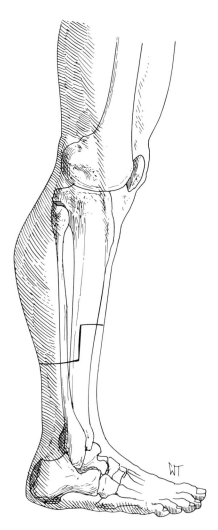

Figure 13-9.   Line of skin incision for the below-knee amputation of the ischemic limb in the coronal plane.

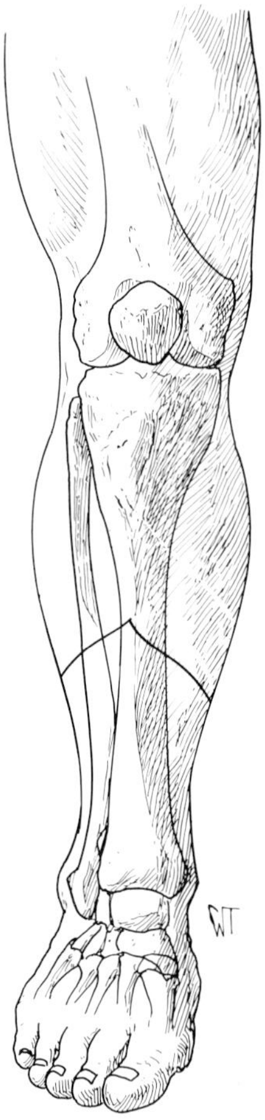

Figure 13-10.   Line of incision for the below-knee amputation of the ischemic limb in the sagittal plane.

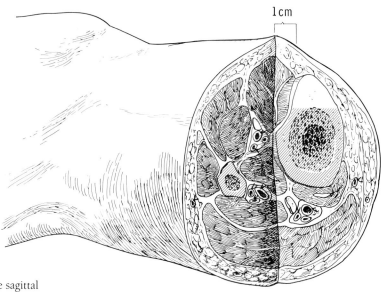

Figure 13-11.   View of the completed amputation in the sagittal plane prior to closure.

lateral flap   medial flap

KNEE DISARTICULATION

Knee disarticulation is indicated when an end-bearing stump is desirable. This is particularly true for the elderly patient; and in some cases, even in patients with peripheral vascular disease.[6] It provides a well-muscled, long stump that often does not need a prosthesis with ischial support. On the other hand, knee disarticulation is contraindicated in an infected leg where an open amputation is necessary. Essential technical details are preservation of skin flaps that are long enough for adequate closure and the preservation of a large area of cancellous bone for weight bearing.[7] The ensuing stump is not cosmetically attractive, and it sometimes presents problems in prosthetic fitting. Supracondylar and high transcondylar amputations fail to provide sufficient weight-bearing surface, so that they become less suitable for end-bearing fitting.

Technique

The patient is placed in the supine position with a sandbag under the pelvis on the affected side to allow for the external rotation of the hip. After suitable preparation and draping and application of the tourniquet, the skin incision is outlined starting 2 cm below the tibial tubercle and then extending toward the crease of the popliteal space of the 90° flexed knee joint (Fig. 13-12). The saphenous vein is ligated, and the saphenous nerve is dissected free and transected well above the level of the incision. The ligamentum patellae is transected as far distally as possible and is raised proximally (Fig. 13-13). Thus the knee joint is entered anteriorly. If possible, the menisci should be left on the femoral side of the stump. This requires transection of the collateral ligament fairly far distally (Fig. 13-14). The cruciate ligaments are resected from the insertion into the tibial plateau. The tendons of the ischiocrural mus-

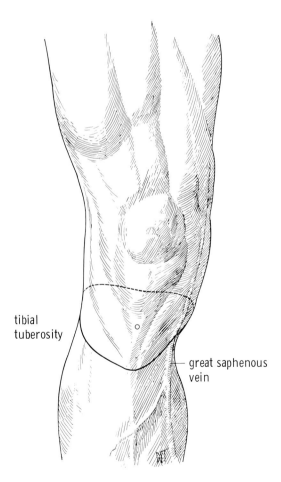

tibial
tuberosity

great saphenous
vein

Figure 13-12.   Line of skin incision for the knee disarticulation.

cles now become accessible. They should be transected as far distally as possible, on the medial side at the pes anserinum, and on the lateral side at the fibular head. With a bone hook, the tibial plateau can now be subluxated forward, and the posterior part of the joint capsule can be transected (Fig. 13-15). Thus, the artery, vein, and nerve in the popliteal space come into view. These are ligated and transected (Fig. 13-16). The nerve should be dissected far enough proximally to stay out of the area of incision. The ligation and transection of the popliteal artery have to be done distally to the branching off of the superior genicular artery. The peroneal nerve has to be transected far enough proximally from the incision.

The patella is now fixed to the patellofemoral joint, either with a cancellous screw or with two threaded Steinmann pins, and with or without denuding the patellofemoral joint of cartilage. The patella tendon is sutured to the stumps of the cruciate ligaments, as are the tendons of the knee flexor muscles (Fig. 13-17). Subcutaneous sutures and skin sutures complete the procedure (Fig. 13-18).

The skin flaps must be long, since retraction of the skin is common, particularly of the posterior part of the thigh. Tightness of the skin over the stump end will lead to circulatory disturbances, and ultimately to breakdown of the stump end. The procedure itself causes very little blood loss.

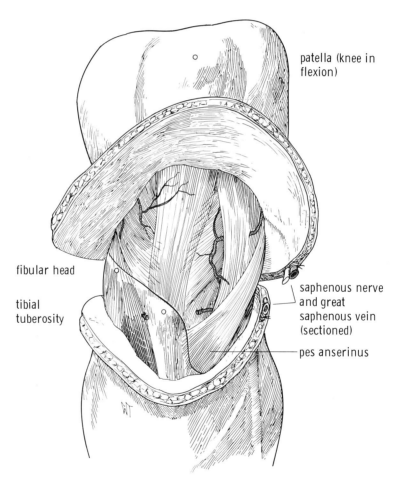

patella (knee in flexion)

fibular head

tibial tuberosity

saphenous nerve and great saphenous vein (sectioned)

pes anserinus

Figure 13-13.   Transection of the patellar ligament and opening of the knee joint capsule.

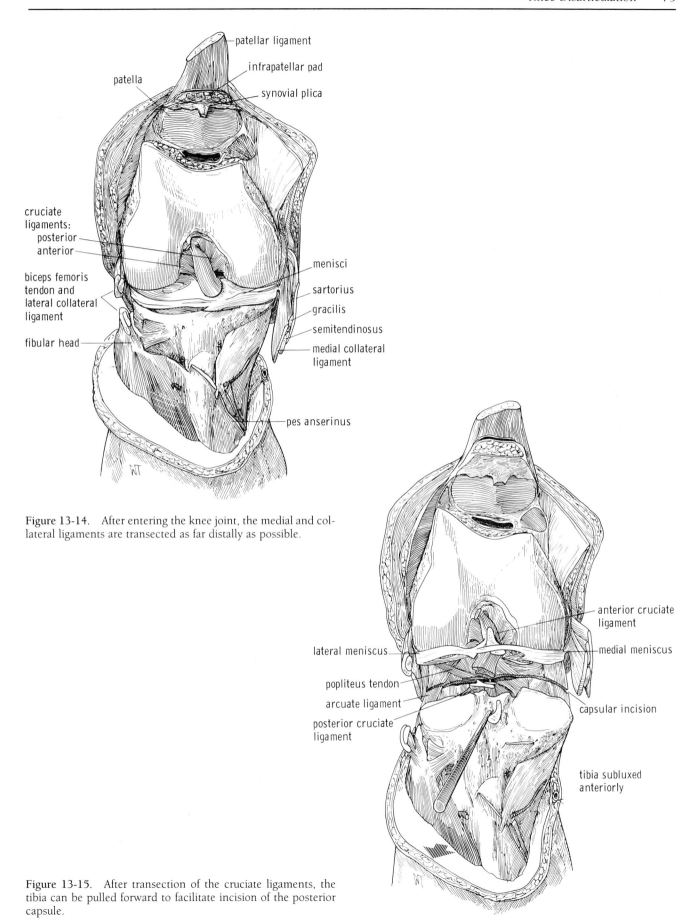

patellar ligament

infrapatellar pad

patella

synovial plica

cruciate
ligaments:
  posterior
  anterior

menisci

biceps femoris
tendon and
lateral collateral
ligament

sartorius

gracilis

semitendinosus

fibular head

medial collateral
ligament

pes anserinus

Figure 13-14.   After entering the knee joint, the medial and col-lateral ligaments are transected as far distally as possible.

anterior cruciate
ligament

lateral meniscus

medial meniscus

popliteus tendon

arcuate ligament

capsular incision

posterior cruciate
ligament

tibia subluxed
anteriorly

Figure 13-15.   After transection of the cruciate ligaments, the tibia can be pulled forward to facilitate incision of the posterior capsule.

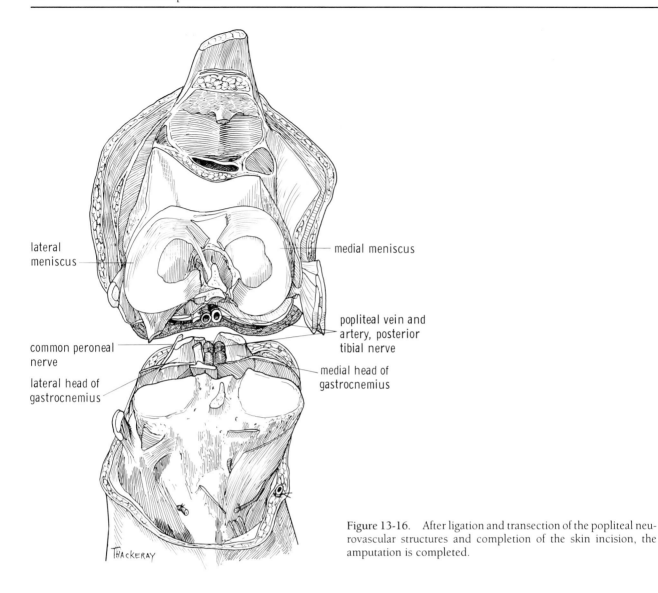

lateral
meniscus

medial meniscus

common peroneal
nerve

popliteal vein and
artery, posterior
tibial nerve

lateral head of
gastrocnemius

medial head of
gastrocnemius

THACKERAY

Figure 13-16. After ligation and transection of the popliteal neurovascular structures and completion of the skin incision, the amputation is completed.

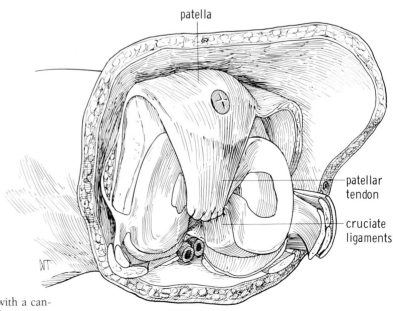

patella

patellar
tendon

cruciate
ligaments

Figure 13-17. The patella is fixed to the condyles with a cancellus screw, and the patellar tendon is sutured to the cruciate ligaments. The meniscii remain on the femoral condyles.

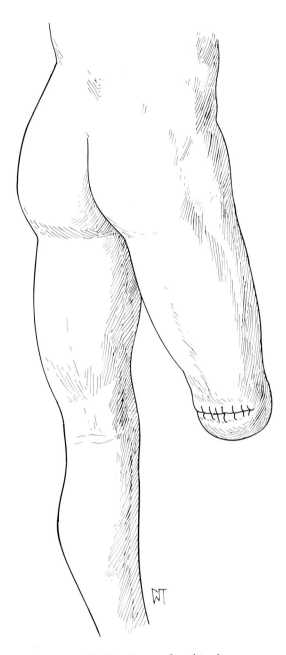

Figure 13-18.   Stump after skin closure.

Modifications

Instead of a tubular opening in the skin, which leads to a longitudinal scar in the intercondylar notch, anterior and posterior flaps either of equal length or with a longer anterior flap can be used. Medial and lateral skin flaps also seem to be durable.

To avoid a bulbous stump end, Mazet and Hennessy in 1966[8,9], recommended removal of the medial half of the medial femoral condyle, the lateral third of the lateral femoral condyle, and the protruding posterior surfaces of both condyles (Fig. 13-19). The patella is excised through a vertical incision in the extensor expansion. The ensuing defect is closed with a running suture. The distal condylar circumference should be 2 to 3 cm greater than the circumference of the amputated thigh in the distal diaphyseal area. The patella tendon is sutured to the cruciate ligaments, the hamstring tendons, and in turn to the extensor expansion. Skin closure is done over a drain.

Burgess[10] later recommended patellectomy and removal of the distal end of the condyles only (Fig. 13-20). Amputation of the leg through the knee is carried out preserving skin flaps of sufficient length, as well as the full length of the cruciate ligament. The menisci are excised. The patella is removed through a vertical incision in the extensor expansion, which is closed with interrupted sutures. The distal ends of the femoral condyles are sawed off parallel to the floor 1.5 cm above the level of the knee joint. The sharp margins of the saw cut are rounded off sparingly with a saw and rasp. The patella tendon is brought into the intercondylar notch and sewn to the stump of the cruciate ligaments (Fig. 13-21). The medial and lateral hamstring tendons are brought forward into the intercondylar notch and sewn to both the extensor expansion and the cruciate ligaments. Closure is achieved over drains.

Knee Disarticulation in Children

The distal femoral epiphysis provides most of the longitudinal growth of the femur. Its preservation in the growing individual is highly desirable. Neither the epiphysis nor the physis should be injured during the surgical procedure. Contouring of the condyles is not necessary. Following the amputation, the distal femoral epiphysis loses its typical formation and, at the end of growth, is smaller and rounder[11]. By the same token, subperiosteal removal of the patella is advisable to avoid pain from chondromalacia.

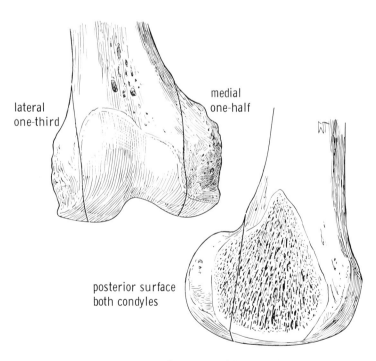

Figure 13-19.   Line of resection of the medial and lateral aspects as well as the posterior aspect of the femoral condyle.

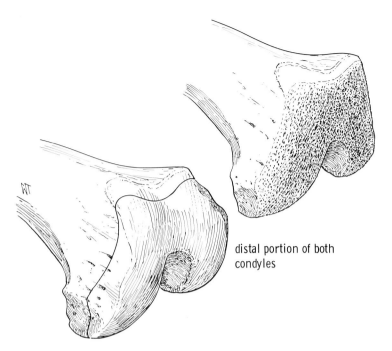

distal portion of both
condyles

Figure 13-20. Resection and rounding of the distal end of the femoral condyles.

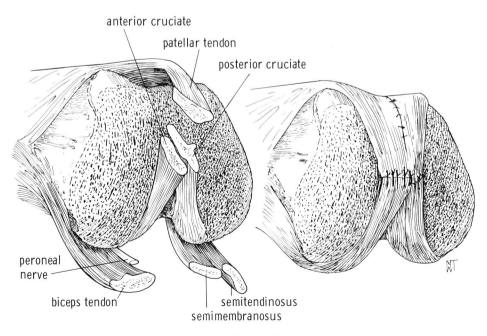

anterior cruciate

patellar tendon

posterior cruciate

peroneal
nerve

biceps tendon

semitendinosus
semimembranosus

Figure 13-21. Attachment of the patellar tendon to the cruciate ligaments and the hamstring tendon.

References

1. Burgess EM, Zettl JH: Amputations below the knee. *Artif Limbs* 13:1–12, 1969.

2. Burgess EM, Romano RL, Zettl JH, Schrock RD: Amputations of the leg for peripheral vascular insufficiency. *J Bone Joint Sur* 53-A: 874–890, 1971.

3. Tracy GD: Below-knee amputation for ischemic gangrene. *Pacific Med Surg* 74:251–253, 1966.

4. Alter AH, Moshein J, Elconin KB, Cohen MJ: Below-knee amputation using the sagittal technique: A comparison with the coronal technique. *Clin Orthopaedics* 131:195–201, 1978.

5. Termansen NB: Below-knee amputation for ischemic gangrene. Prospective, randomized comparison of a transverse and a sagittal operative technique. *Acta Orthop Scand* 48:311–316, 1977.

6. Helmig L: Amputation im Kniegelenk bei Gefässkranken. *Chirurg* 49:228–233, 1978.

7. Baumgartner R: Failures in through-knee amputation. Balgrist Orthopaedic Hospital, University of Zurich. *Prosthetics and Orthotics Int* 7:116–118, 1983.

8. Mazet RJ, Hennessy CA: Knee disarticulation—A new technique and a new knee joint mechanism. *J Bone Joint Surg* 48-A:126–139, 1966.

9. Mazet R Jr, Schmitter ED, Chupurdia R: Disarticulation of the knee. *J Bone Joint Surg* 60-A(5):675–678, 1978.

10. Burgess EM: Disarticulation of the knee. *Arch Surg* 112:1250–1255, 1977.

11. Baumgartner RF: Knee disarticulation versus above-knee amputation. *Prosthetics and Orthotics Int* 3:15–19, 1979.

CHAPTER 14
Above the Knee Amputation

The patient who loses the knee joint mechanism has to exert a considerable amount of energy to work the prosthesis. A knee disarticulation provides the patient with an end-bearing stump. In supracondylar amputations the weight-bearing surfaces that interface with the prosthesis are already away from the end of the stump, and the stump itself becomes the piston that moves the prosthesis. There is, in supracondylar amputations, still a semblance of the distal insertion of the principle thigh muscles if only by suturing the tendons of the flexor and extensor groups together. Those muscles that span the hip joint can forcefully contribute to the active hip movements. The rest are relegated to isometric contractions.

In diaphyseal amputations through the femur, the muscles are transected through the muscle bellies. This makes any attempt at a distal reattachment through myodesis and myoplasty much more tenuous. Some of the muscles lose their innervation and, subsequently, become fibrotic. All of them lose at

least part of their function. The strength of the above-knee amputation stump, therefore, becomes less the shorter it is.

SUPRACONDYLAR AMPUTATIONS

These amputations provide an exceptionally long and usually well-muscled stump. However, their end-bearing properties are not as good as those of the simple or modified knee disarticulation.

Gritti-Stokes Amputation

This amputation provides a stump with the best end-bearing characteristics of the supracondylar computation. It should be considered where knee disarticulation cannot be carried out.[1]

Technique

In the midlateral and midmedial lines, a point at the level of the superior pole of the patella is found. These are the apices of the incision. The inferior pole of the anterior flap is at the tibial tubercle; that of the posterior flap is in the flexor crease of the popliteal fossa. The skin is transected. The patellar tendon is divided at the tibial tubercle and reflected proximally. The muscles in back of the thigh are transected in such a fashion that a slightly beveled surface is achieved. The popliteal vessels are ligated, and the nerves are dissected free and transected well above the level of the incision. The supracondylar area of the femur is transected at a point where its diameter is approximately commensurate to that of the posterior surface of the patella. The posterior surface of the patella itself is removed. Holes are drilled into the distal end of the femoral stump, and also in the remaining anterior part of the patella that remains attached to the quadriceps tendon. Femur and patella are then fitted together in such a fashion that the two bleeding surfaces touch one another. The patella is held in place by number one chromic catgut sutures, which go through corresponding holes in the patella and the femur (Fig. 14-1). The patellar tendon itself can be sutured to the musculature in the back of the femur. The skin is closed in layers after suction drainage has been placed into the wound.

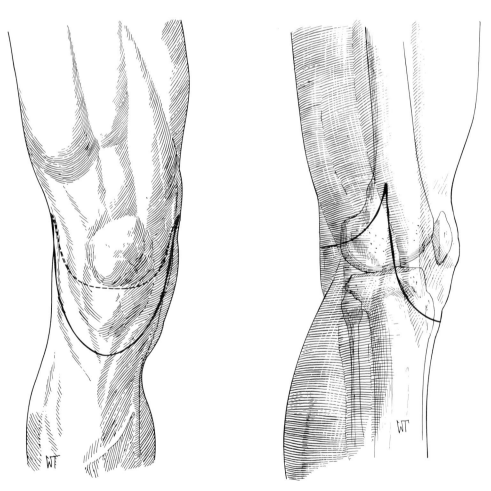

Figure 14-1A.   Skin incision for the Gritti-Stokes amputation.

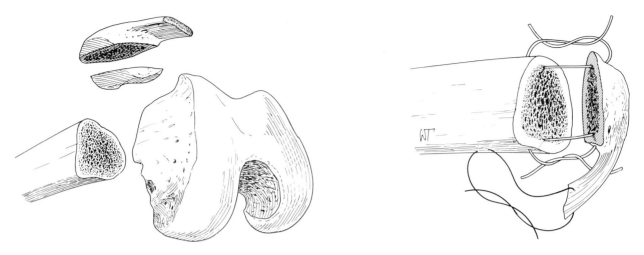

Figure 14-1B.   Schematic outline of the transection of the femur and placement of the anterior part of the patellar over the cut surface in the Gritti-Stokes amputation.

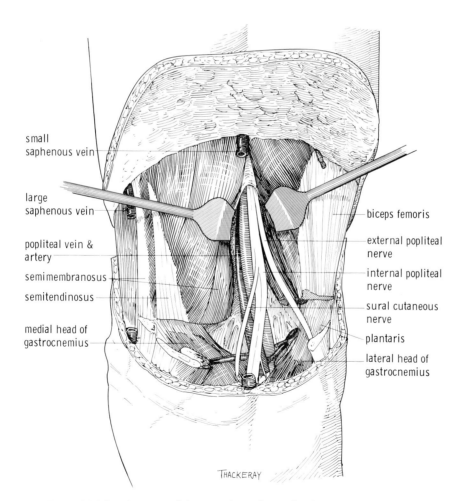

Figure 14-1C.   Anatomy of the area above the popliteal space to be considered in the supracondylar amputations.

Modifications

Slocum recommended a tendoplastic amputation, in which a level slightly lower than the Gritti-Stokes amputation in the proximal end of the flair of the condyles is chosen. The cut surface of the femur is well rounded, and the patella is excised subperiosteally. The soft tissue bed of the patella is then fitted over the distal end of the femur, and the patellar tendon extensor expansion of the knee is sutured to the posterior part of the fascia femoris (Fig. 14-2).

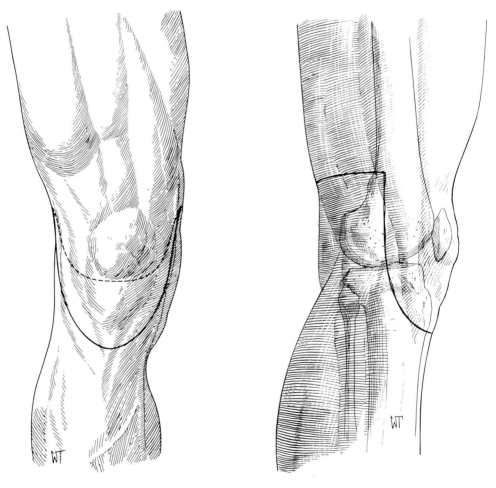

Figure 14-2A.   Skin incision for the Slocum modification of the supracondylar amputation of the femur.

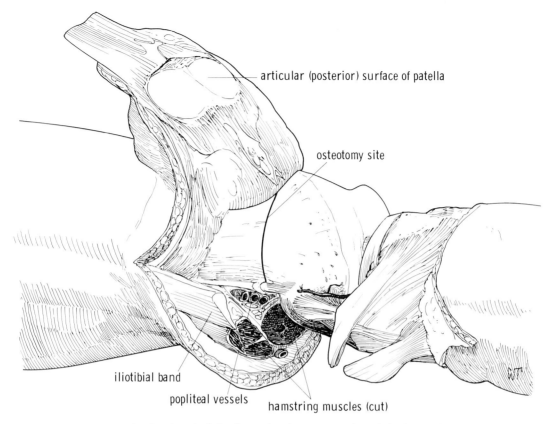

articular (posterior) surface of patella

osteotomy site

iliotibial band

popliteal vessels

hamstring muscles (cut)

Figure 14-2B. The distal end of the femur has been exposed, and the level of transection is indicated.

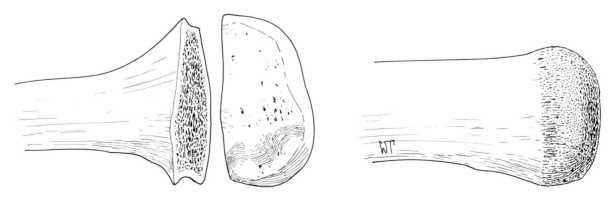

Figure 14-2C. Schematic representation of the shaping of the distal end of the femur.

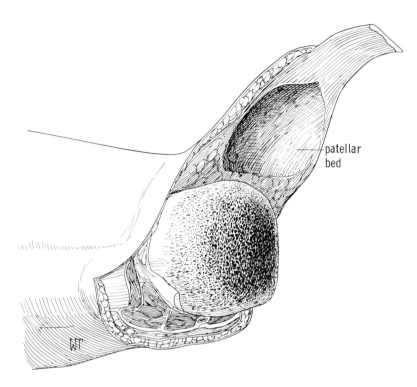

Figure 14-2D.   The patella has been removed and its bed is ready to be approximated to the distal end of the femur.

Callander's Amputation

The creation of a long supracondylar stump and avoidance of transection of muscle fibers are the aims of this procedure. Since the tendons of the knee flexors are not attached to the anterior flap, there is considerable retraction of the posterior skin flap, which leads to positioning of the scar in the back of the stump.

Technique

The patients is placed in the supine position. The knee is flexed approximately 30°. The apex of the incision on the medial side is approximately 5 cm above the adductor tubercle on the lateral side approximately 5 cm above the lateral femoral condyle. The lowest point of the anterior flap is at the tibial tubercle. The posterior flap is of equal length. Medially, the incision is carried through the subcutaneous tissue to the tendons of the medial hamstring muscles, which are transected. After retraction of the proximal tendon stumps, the adductor magnus can be identified with its tendonous attachment to the adductor tubercle of the medial femoral condyle.

It is transected as well. The popliteal space now can be transected free quite easily, and the popliteal vessels and the tibial nerve are ligated and transected.

On the lateral side, the fibers of the iliotibial band have to be split to expose the tendon of the biceps femoris. It is easier to identify the common peroneal nerve from the lateral side, and then to tie it and section it. The posterior incision can now be deepened down to the two heads of the gastrocnemius.

The anterior flap is raised by transecting the patellar tendon, reflecting the quadriceps tendon with the medial and lateral extensor expansion of the quadriceps and the underlying knee joint capsule. The patella is excised subperiosteally. The femoral shaft is exposed up to an area right above the adductor tubercle of the medial femoral condyle. The bone is transected in this area. The anterior and posterior skin flaps are approximated loosely by four to five deep sutures. No attempt is made to secure the free tendon ends.

Following the procedure, the skin flaps are usually very loose. However, the posterior flap has a tendency to retract fairly rapidly, and the anterior flap tightens somewhat over the end of the bony stump. The bed of the patella thus comes to lie over the bony stump end (Fig. 14-3).

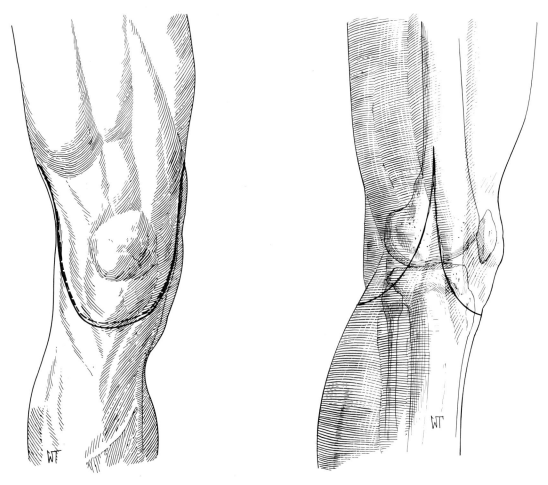

Figure 14-3A.   Skin incision for the Callandar amputation.

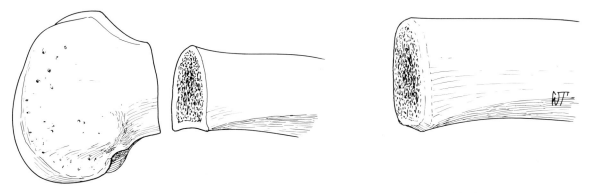

Figure 14-3B.   Schematic representation of the treatment of the distal end of the femur in the Callandar amputation.

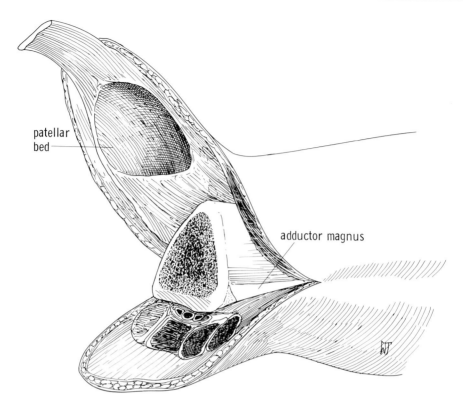

patellar bed

adductor magnus

Figure 14-3C.   The amputation is completed, and the patellar tendon is ready to be approximated to the hamstring musculature.

DIAPHYSEAL AMPUTATION THROUGH THE FEMUR

This type of amputation is the second most common amputation next to the below-knee amputation. In this amputation, the distal attachments of the thigh muscles are lost, and the cylindrical shaft of the femur provides little stability for the thick muscle mass surrounding it that does tend to rotate around it quite freely. On the other hand, good muscle coverage of the stump of the femur is essential for a well-fitting prosthesis, and to the patient's ability to function with a minimum of suspension mechanisms.

Most knee mechanisms extend 8 to 10 cm into the thigh portion of the prosthesis. Thus, a thigh amputation less than 10 cm above the anatomic knee axis may lead to an excessively long stump and unequal knee height. By the same token, a long- well-muscled above-knee stump is desirable, and they should be used where unconventional flaps can prevent an amputation at a higher level.

Technique

With the patient in the supine position, and after suitable preparation and draping, the tourniquet is applied around the upper end of the thigh and inflated (unless there is vascular insufficiency of the leg). In the midmedial and midlateral lines of the thigh, the level of amputation through the shaft of the femur is found. This is the apex of the angle between the anterior and posterior flap (Fig. 14-4). The anterior flap is fashioned distally convex, its length being approximately the sagittal diameter of the thigh. The incision is carried through the subcutaneous tissue and the part of the fascia femoris that lies over the quadriceps. The greatest length of the flap depends on the thickness of the thigh and is between 10 to 20 cm. The posterior flap is slightly shorter. The posterior skin incision is carried through the subcutaneous tissue and the fascia femoris overlying the hamstring muscles. The quadriceps muscle is incised in such a fashion that it bevels back to the intended level of the transection of the femoral shaft. A similar beveling cut is made through the muscle mass of the ischio-crural muscles (Fig. 14-5); however, if the thigh is very muscular, the skin flap is reflected, and the ischiocrural muscles are transected at a point somewhat below the bony transections so they can retract to the level of the bony amputation.

The shaft of the femur is now exposed circumferentially and is transected. Bone shavings are washed away with normal saline, and the veins and arteries are ligated. The femoral artery and vein are found in the femoral canal. The arteria profunda femoris can be found posteriorly to the femoral shaft between the adductor magnus and biceps femoris. The sciatic nerve is identified anteriorly to the hamstring muscles, dissected free well above the level of the bony transection, ligated to avoid bleeding from the arteria concomitans, and then transected. The sensory nerves to the skin are also dissected free and transected (Fig. 14-6). The tourniquet is now released, and hemostasis is obtained.

The wound is closed by approximating the muscle flaps, if these have been fashioned, or by drawing the anterior flap over the end of the bony stump and securing it with interrupted sutures to the fascia at the posterior aspect of the stump.[2] Subcutaneous and interrupted skin sutures are used after a suction drain has been introduced into the wound (Fig. 14-7). Sterile dressings are applied. Since the posterior flap retracts more than the anterior, the incisional scar will ultimately lie behind the level of the bony amputation (Fig. 14-8).

Figures 14-4 to 14-9.   Diaphyseal amputation.

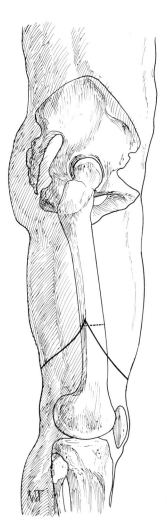

Figure 14-4.   Outline of the skin incision for diaphyseal amputation.

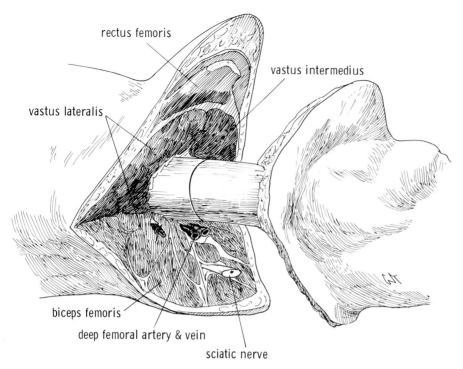

Figure 14-5. Beveling of the anterior and posterior muscle masses.

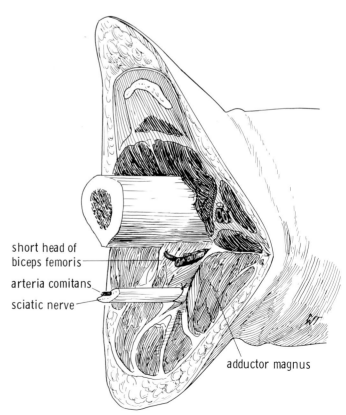

Figure 14-6. Ligation of the blood vessels, and ligation and shortening of the sciatic nerve.

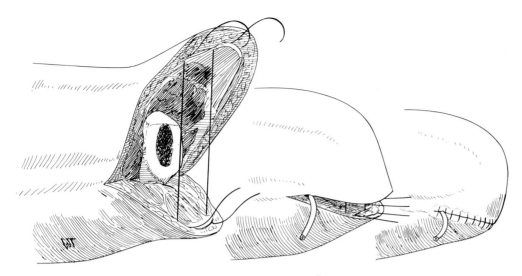

Figure 14-7.   Myoplasty and closure of the amputation wound.

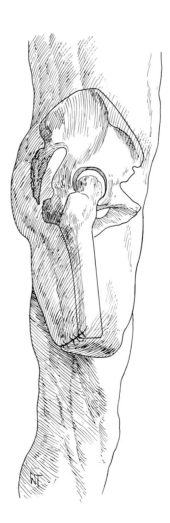

Figure 14-8.   The incision lies at the posterior aspect of the amputation stump.

Alternate Techniques

If no tourniquet is used, it is advisable to dissect free and ligate the major vessels prior to the complete transection of the muscular flaps.

In case myodesis is desirable (Fig. 14-9), four or five holes with a 2.5 mm drill bit are drilled through the cortex at the distal end of the femoral stump.[3]

With 1-0 chromic absorbable sutures, the central layers of the surrounding musculature of the thigh are anchored to the distal end of the femoral stump after the muscles themselves have been put under tension. This is particularly advisable where a long anterior quadriceps flap is used to cover the stump end.

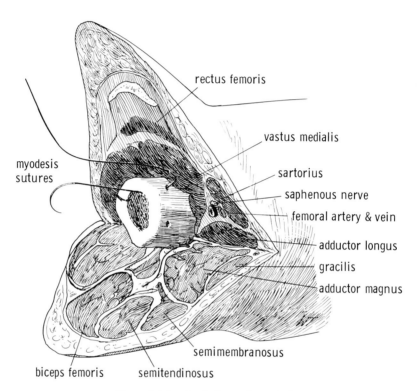

Figure 14-9.   Technique of myodesis.

ABOVE-KNEE AMPUTATION IN CHILDREN

The distal femoral epiphysis contributes approximately 70% to the longitudinal growth of the femur. The earlier amputation through the femur has been carried out in a child, the more the remnant of the femur will lag behind in growth and development. By comparison, the soft tissue coverage around the femur lags behind much less, so that at the end of growth, a very fleshy stump often results with little skeletal scaffolding. Indeed, symptomatic bony overgrowth is very rare in diaphyseal amputation of the femur in the child.

Even in disarticulation of the knee in early childhood, considerable retardation of growth has to be expected. In addition to that, altered muscle stresses around the hip joint lead to a retardation in the development of the acetabulum, which may result in the subluxation of the hip joint on the affected side.[4]

Therefore, while the technical details of the amputation through the thigh of the child do not substantially differ from that of the adult, the later growth and development should be kept in mind. The longer the remainder of the femur, the more of a thigh stump can be expected. Particularly in the young child, when disarticulation at the knee is possible, it is highly preferable to a diaphyseal amputation.

TURN-UP PLASTY OF THE LEG

In cases where there is a normal or near-normal hip joint and trochanteric region and a normal lower leg, and where resection of the subtrochanteric part of the femur becomes necessary, turn-up plasty of the leg may be a reasonable alternative to hip disarticulation.[5,6] This procedure is also possible for the formation of an above-knee stump in cases where the femoral diaphysis has been destroyed by infection. Indeed, attempts have been made to implant the lateral malleolus to the acetabulum in an attempt to create a new hip joint where resection of the entire femur has become necessary. The principle of the procedure is to preserve all major blood vessels and nerves, as well as the muscles powering the hip. The turning up of the leg can be done in the sagittal, as well as coronal planes. The choice of the direction of the turn-up is dictated by the area of skin and muscle that has to be resected. If complete turn-up plasty is planned, the coronal plane has to be chosen by necessity.

Partial Turn-Up Plasty

Temporary hemostasis can be obtained by inserting a Steinmann pin above the greater trochanter and using an Esmarch bandage as a tourniquet through the perineum. The patient is in lateral position, lying on the sound side. A 12- to 15-cm wide strip of skin is removed from the lateral aspect of the lower extremity (Fig. 14-10). The underlying soft tissue is resected according to the needs. If a malignant tumor is resected, sufficient soft tissue must be maintained around it, so as not to breach the integrity of the tumor. It is, however, of utmost importance to maintain the vessels on the medial and posterior sides of the thigh and the sciatic nerve. The proximal end of the femur is amputated subtrochanterically, leaving sufficient amounts of bone for a stable osteosynthesis (Fig. 14-11). The distal end of the femur is disarticulated at the level of the knee (Fig. 14-12).

Scar tissue is resected in such a way that a well vascularized bed is prepared to receive the bones of the lower leg (Fig. 14-13).

On the lateral aspect of the leg, sufficient musculature from the lateral and posterior compartment must be sacrificed to avoid excess bulk when the lower leg is turned up into the thigh region. The fibula may have to be removed, preserving the interosseous vessels. The foot and lower part of the leg are amputated according to the length of the stump desired. Sauerbruch[7] recommended the insertion of an intermedullary dowel shaped from the fibula to unite the proximal end of the femur to the distal end of the tibia. Otherwise, osteosynthesis with plate and screw has to be performed. The tourniquet, if any, is removed, and meticulous hemostasis is obtained. The lower part of the leg is then turned up in a coronal plane into the bed prepared in the thigh, and the distal end of the tibia is united to the proximal end of the femur (Fig. 14-14). Several suction drains are inserted into the wound and the wound is closed in layers (Fig. 14-15).

Postoperatively, it is best to maintain the patient in a hip spica for two weeks. Following removal of the spica, active range of motion exercises should be initiated.

Where excision of the entire femur becomes necessary, an attempt can be made to use the lateral malleolus as a means of counterpressure as it is inserted into the acetabulum. The turn-up in this case has to be done in the coronal plane, so that the lateral malleolus ends up on the medial side of the ankle joint. The approach is the same as previously described. When excision of the femur is required in the adult, approximately 4 to 5 cm of the proximal end of the tibia has to be sacrificed. In the child, in an attempt to preserve the proximal tibial and fibular epiphyses, diaphyseal-shortening osteotomy may become necessary to allow turn-up of the lower leg without excessive tension on the skin at the distal end of the stump. Alternatively, a total hip arthroplasty can be performed (Fig. 14-16).

The capsule of the ankle joint should be preserved, and an attempt should be made to attach it to the remnants of the hip capsule. The tendons of the abductor muscles can be inserted into the deltoid ligament around the medial malleolus (Fig. 14-17). A tibiofibular synostosis at the proximal end of the ankle becomes necessary.

If scarring is excessive in the anterior aspect of the lower extremity, the turn-up can be performed as originally described by Sauerbruch[7] in the sagittal plane. This would then require excision of the scarred area in the anterior aspect of the thigh and excision of an equally wide strip of skin and soft tissue from the anterior aspect of the lower leg. The amputation of the femur is done through this anterior approach. The amputation of the foot and the lower part of he leg are done in a guillotine fashion (Fig. 14-18).

Figures 14-10 to 14-18.   Turn-up plasty.

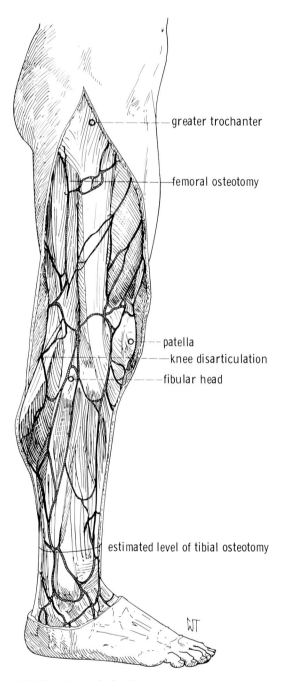

Figure 14-10.   Removal of a skin strip from the lateral aspect of the lower extremity.

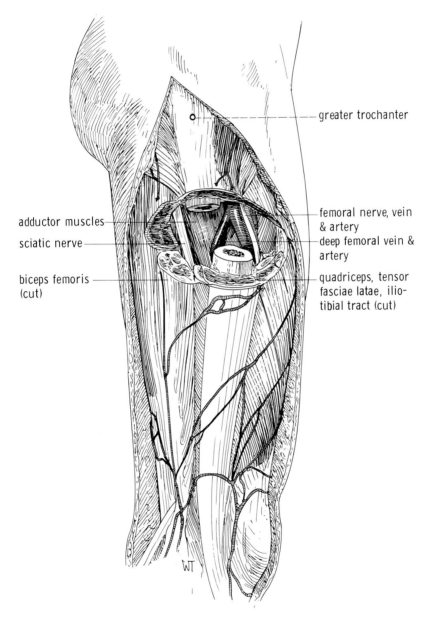

greater trochanter

femoral nerve, vein & artery

adductor muscles

sciatic nerve

deep femoral vein & artery

biceps femoris (cut)

quadriceps, tensor fasciae latae, iliotibial tract (cut)

Figure 14-11. Exposure and transection of the subtrochanteric area of the femur.

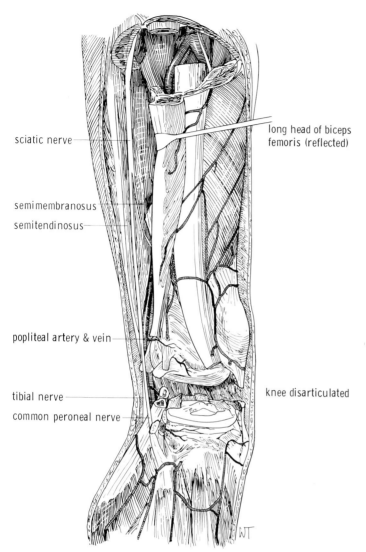

sciatic nerve

long head of biceps
femoris (reflected)

semimembranosus

semitendinosus

popliteal artery & vein

tibial nerve

common peroneal nerve

knee disarticulated

Figure 14-12.   Disarticulation at the knee.

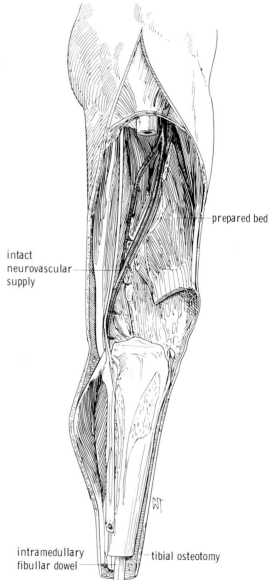

prepared bed

intact
neurovascular
supply

intramedullary
fibullar dowel

tibial osteotomy

Figure 14-13.   The soft tissue bed in the thigh has been prepared,
and the tibia is ready for the turn-up.

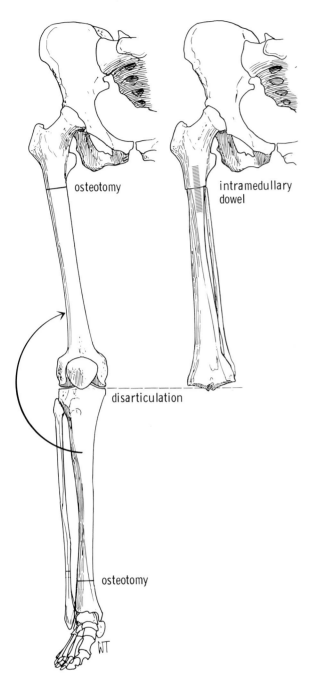

osteotomy

intramedullary
dowel

disarticulation

osteotomy

WT

Figure 14-14.   Schematic representation of the turn-up plasty in
the coronal plane.

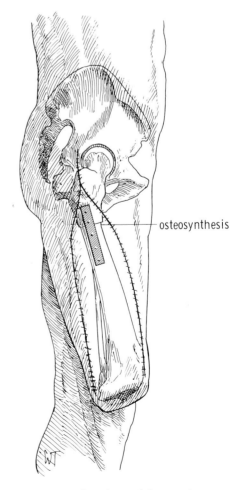

osteosynthesis

WT

Figure 14-15.   Skin closure following the turn-up.

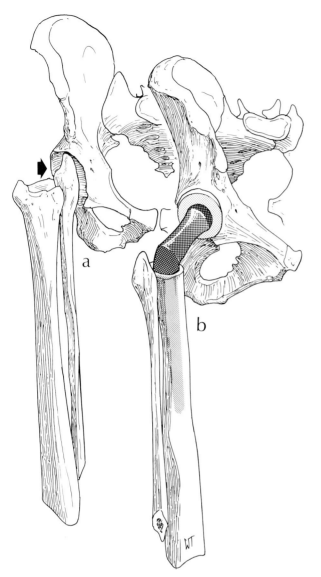

Figure 14-16.   a. Maintenance of the lateral malleolus to be placed into the acetabulum. b. Total hip arthroplasty as an alternate method of hip reconstruction.

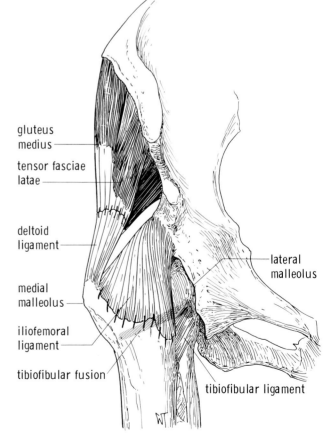

gluteus medius

tensor fasciae latae

deltoid ligament

medial malleolus

iliofemoral ligament

tibiofibular fusion

lateral malleolus

tibiofibular ligament

Figure 14-17.   Tibiofibular fusion and attachment of remnants of the hip capsule to the ankle capsule.

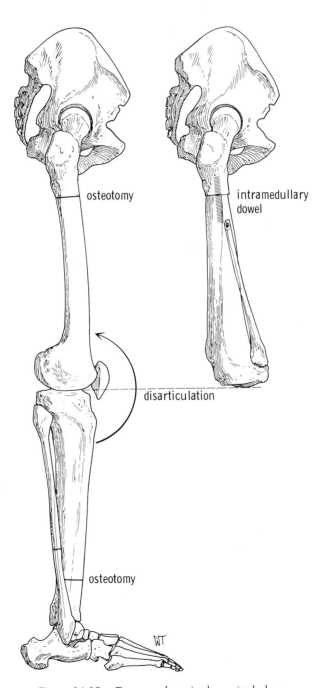

Figure 14-18.   Turn-up plasty in the sagittal plane.

TURNAROUND PLASTY

Borggreve-van Ness Rotational Osteotomy[8,9]

Among the intercalary amputations, the rotational osteotomy of the lower extremity has gained increasing acceptance. It is used for the construction of a knee joint out of the ankle joint by rotating the lower extremity through an osteotomy, through an arch of 180°, and at the same time shortening it sufficiently. The procedure has been used for en bloc resections of tumors at the lower end of the femur, as well as in the care of a patient with proximal femoral focal deficiency. In the latter case, knee fusion can be done if necessary at the same time, and the incision through the knee can be used to aid in the rotation of the lower extremity.

The contraindication in the case of the tumor patient is clear. The tumor must be resectable en bloc, and without being exposed even during the exposure of the nerves and blood vessels. In the patient with femoral focal deficiency, the deformity must be unilateral. The rotated ankle should ultimately be approximately at the level of the knee joint on the sound side. There must be a good range of dorsiflexion and plantarflexion in the ankle actively and passively before surgery, and the muscle power around the ankle should be near normal. While fibular hypoplasia or absence of the fibula need not be a contraindication, deformities of the foot are. Indeed, nothing should be done to weaken the foot. Amputations of the toes should be avoided.

Complications of the rotational osteotomy include ischemia in the rotated part of the leg, nonunion of the osteotomy site, and re-rotation of the lower extremity with poor alignment of the new "knee joint." For the last reason, it is not advisable to do the rotational osteotomy on any patient younger than 12 years.

Technique in the Nontumor Patient[10,11]

The patient is in a supine position (Fig. 14-19). Anesthesia is induced, and the tourniquet is inflated. The skin incision is over the anterior aspect of the leg either vertical, approximately 1 cm lateral of the tibial crest, or oblique from medially proximal to laterally distal. The tibial diaphysis is exposed subperiosteally, and a section of about 8 or 9 cm are marked for resection. Proximally and distally to the limits of the bone to be dissected, two landmarks are created by shallow drill holes. This will ensure an adequate amount of rotation at the end of the procedure. The fibula is now exposed subperiosteally, and a section slightly longer than the one resected from the tibial diaphysis is resected from the fibular diaphysis. The tourniquet is now released, and accurate hemostasis is obtained.

A section of the fibular diaphysis is fashioned to act as an intermedullary peg for the tibia. It is inserted into the proximal end of the marrow cavity. The distal end of the leg is now rotated 180°. During this procedure, the circulation in the foot has to be observed closely to avoid ischemia. The marrow cavity of the distal end of the tibia is now impaled on the peg at the proximal end of the tibia. Kirschner wires are inserted horizontally into the two fragments of the tibia. They are maintained in an external fixation device. Skin closure only is carried out. The lower extremity is maintained in a soft, bulky dressing. The sole of the foot and the toes are left free for inspection.

Technique in the Patient with a Malignant Tumor at the Distal End of the Femur[12,13]

The surgical procedure is changed to allow en bloc resection (Fig. 14-20). The incision allows removal of a romboid of skin, which in its long axis is approximately 5 cm longer than the overall length of the planned subcutaneous resection. Then a longitudinal extension of the incision 8 cm distally from the distal angle of the romboid is added (Fig. 14-21). The peroneal nerve is exposed and traced proximally to expose the bifurcation of the sciatic nerve. The tibial nerve and the femoral and popliteal vessels are exposed distally from the adductor canal onward (Fig. 14-22). All branches into the area of planned resection have to be ligated and cut. Distally, the muscles are cut at the level of the intended transection of the bone. Proximally, the muscles are transected 5 cm above the level of transection of the femur. Two transverse Kirschner wires are inserted parallel to one another into the proximal fragment of the femur and the distal fragment of the tibia (Fig. 14-23). The bone is transected, and the resected area — including the tumor — is lifted out of the wound. The gap in the lower extremity is bridged only by neurovascular structures (Fig. 14-24).

The lower end of the lower extremity is rotated 180°. A notch is cut into the posterior aspect of the tibia to receive the proximal end of the femur. Osteosynthesis between tibia and femur is achieved with plate and screws. There is now considerable slack and tortuosity in the neurovascular bundle (Fig. 14-25).

The aponeurosis of the quadriceps and its tendon are sutured to the triceps muscle at the calf. The toe extensors are sutured to the hamstring tendons (Fig. 14-26). During these steps in the procedure, care has to be taken not to obstruct the blood flow. The circulation in the foot must be observed closely. Because of the oblique orientation of the skin incision, skin closure is usually not difficult despite the difference in circumference of the two segments of the remainder of the limb (Fig. 14-27).

With stable osteosynthesis, the Kirschner wires can be removed, and a soft dressing can be applied.

Figures 14-19 to 14-27.   Turnaround plasty.

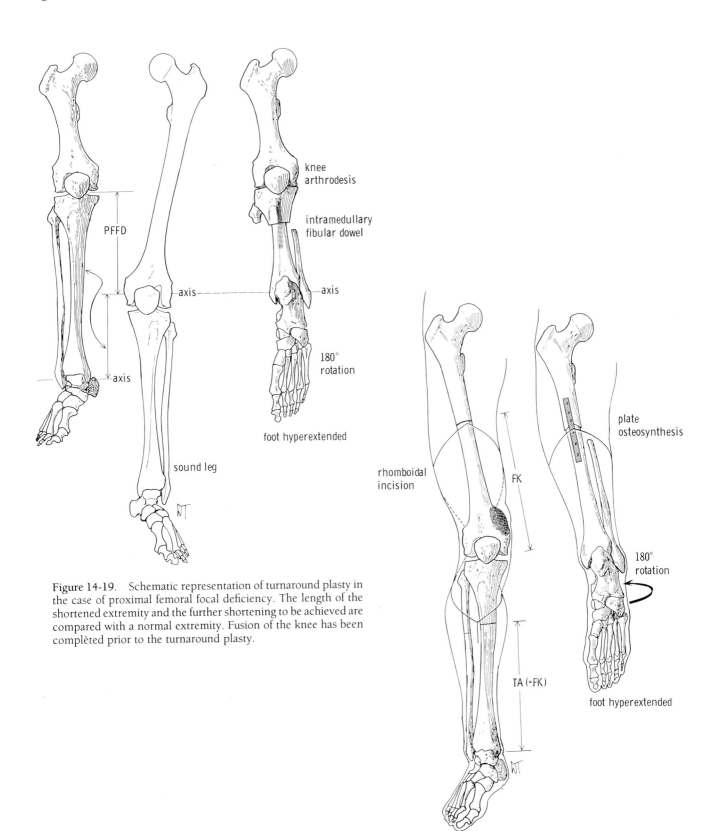

knee
arthrodesis

intramedullary
fibular dowel

axis

180°
rotation

foot hyperextended

sound leg

PFFD

axis

axis

Figure 14-19.   Schematic representation of turnaround plasty in the case of proximal femoral focal deficiency. The length of the shortened extremity and the further shortening to be achieved are compared with a normal extremity. Fusion of the knee has been completed prior to the turnaround plasty.

rhomboidal
incision

FK

plate
osteosynthesis

180°
rotation

foot hyperextended

TA (=FK)

Figure 14-20.   Schematic representation of turnaround plasty in the case of a tumor patient.

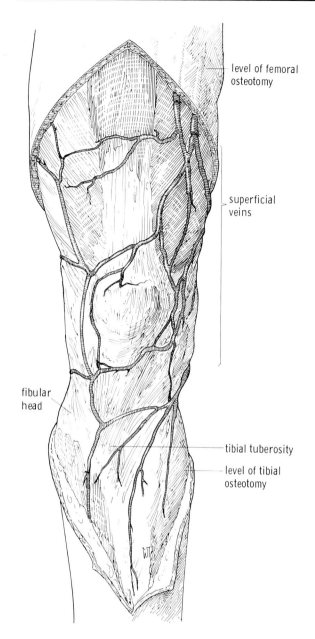

Figure 14-21.   Romboid skin incision.

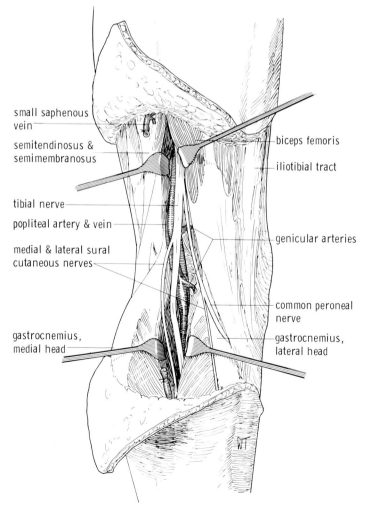

Figure 14-22.   Exposure of the neurovascular bundle.

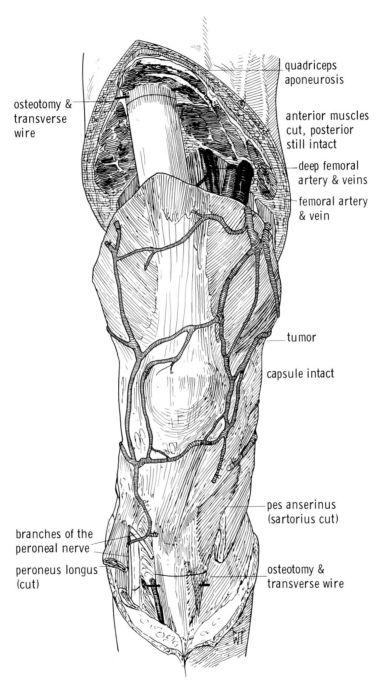

osteotomy &
transverse
wire

quadriceps
aponeurosis

anterior muscles
cut, posterior
still intact

deep femoral
artery & veins

femoral artery
& vein

tumor

capsule intact

pes anserinus
(sartorius cut)

branches of the
peroneal nerve

peroneus longus
(cut)

osteotomy &
transverse wire

Figure 14-23.   Exposure of tibia and femur after transection of the soft
tissues. Insertion of the Kirschner wires as markers.

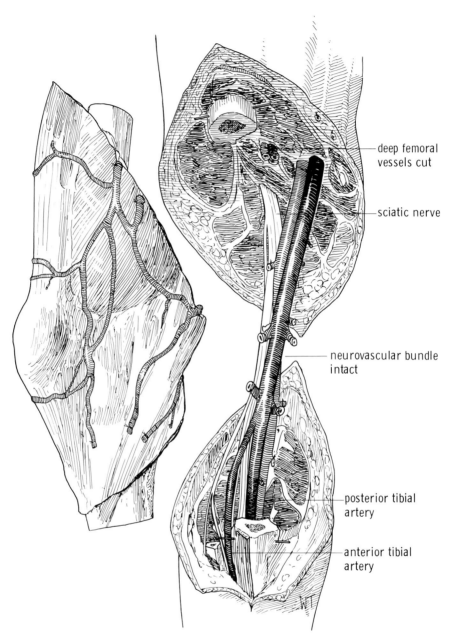

deep femoral
vessels cut

sciatic nerve

neurovascular bundle
intact

posterior tibial
artery

anterior tibial
artery

Figure 14-24.   After removal of the en bloc resected tumor, the defect in the lower
extremity is bridged by the neurovascular structures only.

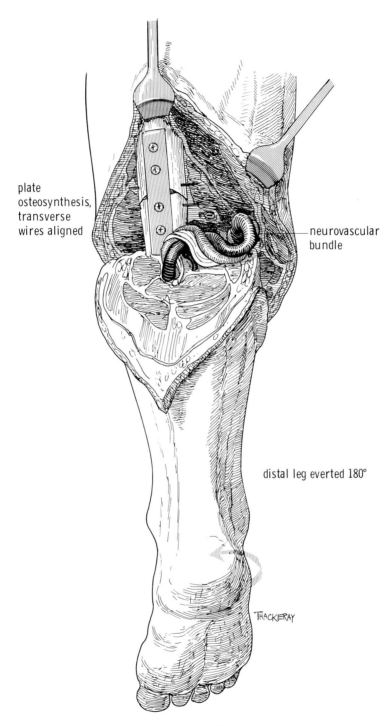

plate
osteosynthesis,
transverse
wires aligned

neurovascular
bundle

distal leg everted 180°

THACKERAY

Figure 14-25.   Osteosynthesis has been completed.

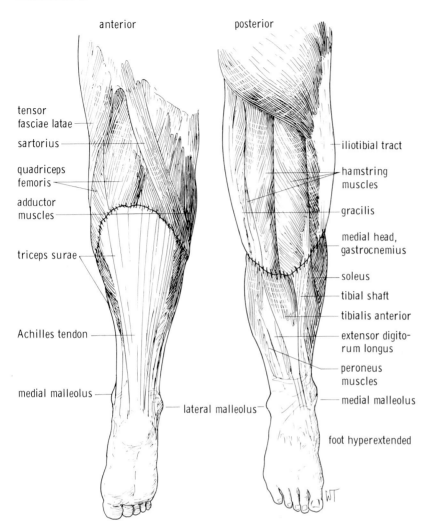

Figure 14-26.   Reconstitution of muscular integrity.

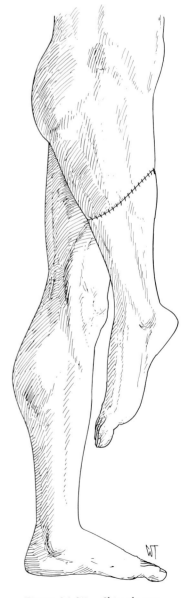

Figure 14-27.   Skin closure.

DISARTICULATION OF THE HIP[14]

Technique

To determine the incision for hip disarticulation, it is best to outline the anterior superior iliac spine, the inguinal ligament, and a circular line around the thigh approximately 5 cm below the pubic tubercle and the ischial tuberosity. The incision itself is a racquet incision (Fig. 14-28), starting medial to and below the anterior superior iliac spine and running down parallel to the inguinal ligament toward the midmedial line of the thigh, where it meets the circumferential line around the thigh. It is continued around the posterior aspect of the thigh, and starts to gently curve up in the midlateral line of the thigh toward the starting point of the incision. Through the anterior part of the incision, the femoral artery and vein are isolated and ligated (Fig. 14-29). The femoral nerve is dissected free and followed toward the inguinal ligament, where it is ligated and transected. The muscles originating from the superior and inferior anterior iliac spines are detached at their origin and held downward. Now the pectineus muscle comes into view. It is transected a finger breadth away from the pubis ramus. By externally rotating the hip, the lesser trochanter can be brought into view and the iliopsoas tendon can be transected at its insertion here. Adductor and gracilis muscles are being detached from the pubic bone, and the adductor magnus is transected as it originates from the ischium.

Between the pectineus and external rotators of the hip, the obturator artery and its branches can be identified and ligated. Care has to be taken to transect the obturator externus well away from the obturator foramen (Fig. 14-29), as the obturator artery can be transected inadvertently in this region. It then retracts into the lesser pelvis, and great difficulties can be encountered in recovering its cut end for ligation.

By internal rotation of the hip (Fig. 14-30), the greater trochanter can be identified and the gluteus medius and minimus can be detached from their insertions into the greater trochanter. These muscles are retracted upward. The fascia lata is divided either above or below the insertion of the tensor fasciae latae in the line of the skin incision. In its posterior aspect, the lower fibers of the gluteus maximus are divided as well, and the tendon of the gluteus maximus is detached from its insertion into the linea aspera. Now the sciatic nerve can be identified, dissected free, ligated, and divided as far proximally as possible. If the external rotators of the hip have not been transected thus far, they can be divided at this point. This gives access to the hamstring muscles at the ischial tuberosity, which are divided at their origin. The femur is now held only by its attachments through the capsule and the intra-articular ligament, which are transected closely to the acetabulum (Fig. 14-31). The femoral head is then dislocated.

Closure of the wound is accomplished by bringing the gluteus medius and minimus over the acetabulum and suturing them into the transverse ligament (Fig. 14-32). A suction drain is placed into the wound, and the gluteus maximus is brought forward and downward and sutured into the origin of the pectineus muscle and the adductors (Fig. 14-33). Another drain should be placed subcutaneously into the lower part of the incision. The skin should be sutured without any tension (Figs. 14-34 and 14-35).

Posteromedial Flap Coverage

If removal of the entirety of the lateral part of the thigh becomes desirable, posteromedial flaps offer adequate coverage of the gluteal musculature. The skin incision starts over the lacuna vasorum at the level of the inguinal ligament, follows the femoral artery approximately 10 cm distally, turns medially and posteriorly, and continues posterolaterally and laterally to the tip of the greater trochanter and further to its point of origin. The femoral vessels are isolated and ligated. The femoral nerve is dissected free, to be pulled gently into the wound, ligated, and transected in such a way that it retracts beyond the iguinal ligament. Both the sartorius from the anterior superior iliac spine and the rectus femoris from the inferior iliac spine are resected; the tensor fascia latae muscle is removed either from its origin at the pelvis or transected at the level of the skin incision. Laterally, the abductor muscles are visualized and transected at their insertion into the greater trochanter.

Medially, the adductor muscles are resected from their origin at the tuberculum pubis. Both branches of the obturtor nerve are dissected free, and then transected as far proximally as possible. Further abducting the hip, the origin of the adductors from the pubic ramus is transected. One must take care to ligate the obturtor artery prior to transection, since it has a tendency to retract into the obturator foramen and is difficult to ligate thereafter. The ischiocrural muscles are then transected at their origin at the ischial bone. The gluteus maximus is transected at the level of the skin incision, and the sciatic nerve is dissected free, ligated, and transected. The capsule of the hip joint can now be incised, and the disarticulation is completed.

The insertion of the gluteus medius and minimus can be sutured into the transverse acetabular ligament after a drain has been inserted below them. The drain is brought into the wound, and the muscle flap of the gluteus maximus is brought forward and medially to the pubic ramus and tuberculum pubis. It is sutured into the remaining periosteum. The skin edges are trimmed, and a third drain is placed into the inferior part of the incision before the skin edges are sutured.

If dissection of the deep iliac lymph nodes becomes desirable,[15] a vertical limb at the starting point of the incision over the inguinal ligament of 4 or 5 cm is added. Two skin flaps medially and laterally can be developed, and the subcutaneous tissue over the inguinal region and the abdominal wall can be dissected. The entire inguinal region, including the iguinal canal, is denuded. The inguinal ligament is incised and retracted. Through this entrance into the retroperitoneal space, the iliac vessels can be followed proximally; areolar tissue as well as lymph nodes from the vessels can be dissected. To this end, the peritoneum and bladder are being retracted medially. If further exposure is required, the abdominal muscles can be incised further.

Figures 14-28 to 14-35.   Disarticulation of the hip.

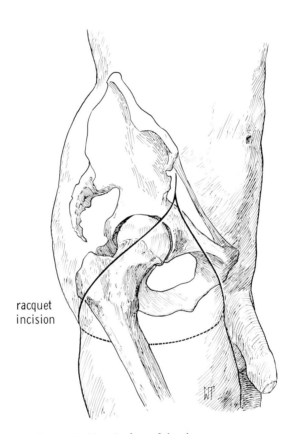

Figure 14-28.   Outline of the skin incision.

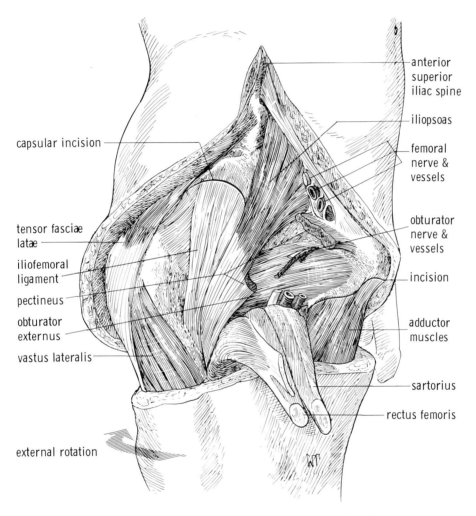

anterior
superior
iliac spine

iliopsoas

femoral
nerve &
vessels

obturator
nerve &
vessels

incision

adductor
muscles

sartorius

rectus femoris

capsular incision

tensor fasciae
latae

iliofemoral
ligament

pectineus

obturator
externus

vastus lateralis

external rotation

Figure 14-29.   Exposure of the anterior, anteromedial, and lateral structures.

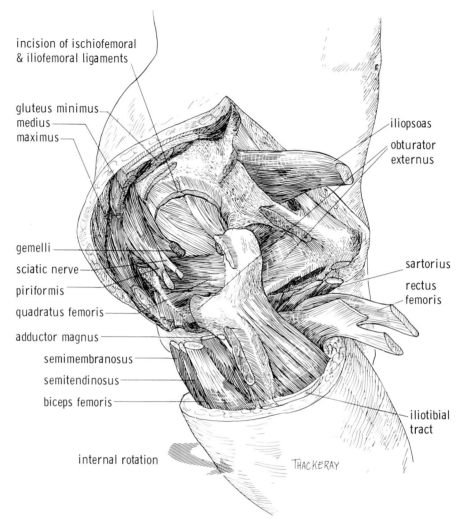

incision of ischiofemoral
& iliofemoral ligaments

gluteus minimus
medius
maximus

iliopsoas

obturator
externus

gemelli

sciatic nerve

piriformis

quadratus femoris

adductor magnus

semimembranosus

semitendinosus

biceps femoris

sartorius

rectus
femoris

iliotibial
tract

internal rotation

THACKERAY

Figure 14-30.   Transection of the posterolateral and posterior structures.

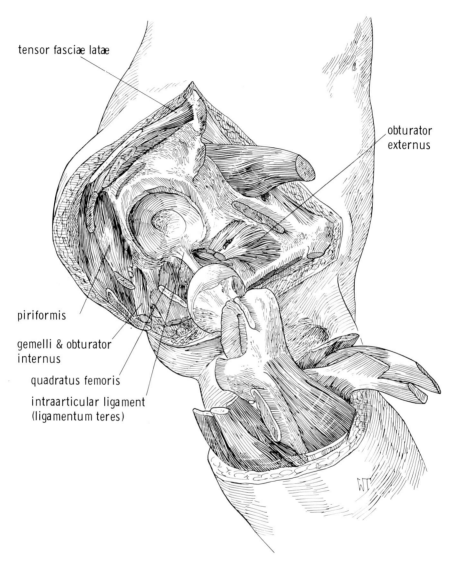

tensor fasciæ latæ

obturator
externus

piriformis

gemelli & obturator
internus

quadratus femoris

intraarticular ligament
(ligamentum teres)

Figure 14-31.   Femoral head has been disarticulated and is only held by the ligamentum teres.

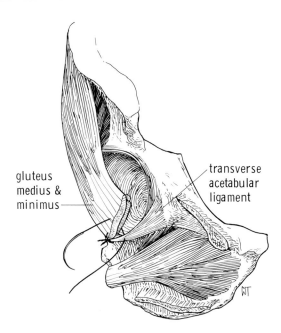

Figure 14-32. Gluteus medius and minimus are used for coverage of the acetabulum.

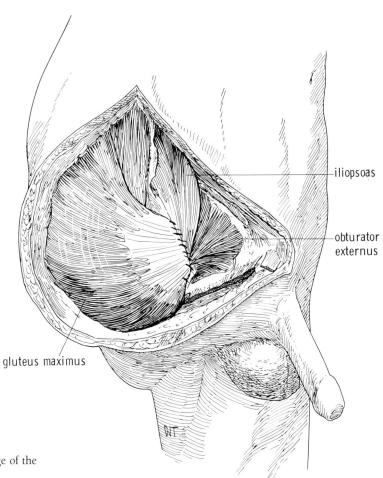

Figure 14-33. The gluteus maximus is used for coverage of the posterolateral aspect of the pelvis.

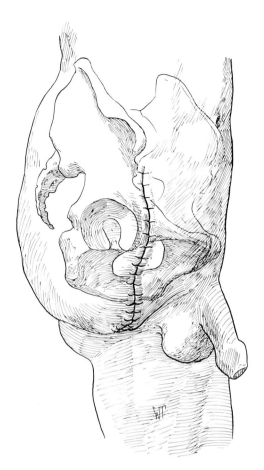

Figure 14-34. Skin closure.

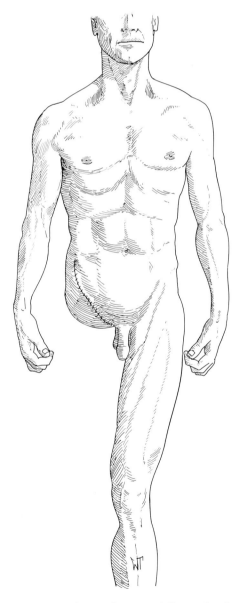

Figure 14-35. Frontal view of a patient following hip disarticulation.

References

1. Doran J, Hopkinson BR, Makin GS: The Gritti-Stokes amputation in ischaemia: A review of 134 cases. *Br J Surg* 65:135–137, 1978.

2. Weiss M (ed): *Myoplastic Amputation, Immediate Prosthesis and Early Ambulation.* US Department of Health, Education, and Welfare, Washington, DC, 1971.

3. Burgess EM, Romano RL, Zettl JD: *The Management of Lower Extremity Amputations.* Veterans Administration, Washington, DC, TR 10-6, 1969.

4. Baumgartner RF: Above-knee amputation in children. *Prosthetics and Orthotics Int* 3:26–30, 1979.

5. Van Nes CP: "Turn-up plasty" of the leg. *J Bone Joint Surg* 30-A:854–858, 1948.

6. Thompson TC: Turn-up plasty amputation. *Maryland State Med J* 5:673–674, 1956.

7. Sauerbruch F: Die Exstirpation des Femur mit Um-kipp-Plastic des Unterschenkels. *Deutsche Zeitschrift für Chirurgie* 163:1–12, 1922.

8. Borggreve J: Kniegelenksersatz durch das in der Bein-längsachse um 180° gedrehte Fussgelenk. *Arch Orthop Unfall Chir* 28:175–178, 1930.

9. Van Nes CP: Rotation-plasty for congenital defects of the femur. *J Bone Joint Surg* 32-B:12–16, 1950.

10. Kostuik JP, Gillespie R, Hall JE, Hubbard S: Van Nes rotational osteotomy for treatment of proximal femoral focal deficiency and congenital short femur. *J Bone Joint Surg* 57-A:1039–1046, 1975.

11. Kritter AE: Tibial rotation-plasty for proximal femoral focal deficiency. *Bone Joint Surg* 59-A:927–933, 1977.

12. Salzer M, Knahr K: Resection of malignant bone tumors. *Recent Res Cancer Res* 54:239–255, 1976.

13. Salzer M, Knahr K, Kotz R, Kirsten H: Treatment of osteosarcomata of the distal femur by rotation-plasty. *Arch Orthopaedic Traumatic Surg* 99:131–136, 1981.

14. Boyd HB: Anatomic disarticulation of the hip. *Surg Gynecol Obstet* 84:346–349, 1947.

15. Pack GT, Ehrlich HE: Exarticulation of the lower extremities for malignant tumors: Hip joint disarticulation (with and without deep iliac dissection) and sacroiliac disarticulation (hemipelvectomy). *Ann Surg* 123:965–985, 1946.

CHAPTER 15
Hemipelvectomy

Removal of half of the pelvic girdle is done almost exclusively for eradication of malignant tumors of both the proximal end of the lower extremity and the hemipelvis. Occasionally, overwhelming infections at the proximal end of the lower extremity, such as gas gangrene, may require hemipelvectomy. Being extremely mutilating, hemipelvectomy adds to the physical trauma a severe psychological stress. The patient comes to realize in the days and weeks following the operation that he has lost what he considers to be one-fourth of his or her body. The patient will need considerable psychological support during the postoperative period to help carry this burden. At the same time, the hemipelvectomy has, without any question, improved the long-term survival of patients with malignant tumors close to the trunk. Therefore, when proposing the procedure, all details should be fully explained and no doubt should be left as to the probable consequence of inadequate compromises.

PREPARATION

The preoperative preparation of the patient includes antibiotic treatment or at least suppression of any infection that may be present. The patient should be in good physical condition prior to the surgery. However, if a patient does not have an adequate blood count prior to surgery, he or she should at least be started on a transfusion at the beginning of surgery, since large blood loss is to be expected. On the evening before surgery, a cleansing enema should be given, and the patient needs an indwelling urethral catheter as well as a nasogastric tube during and after surgery.[1,2]

Before starting the actual surgical procedure, an intravenous pressure catheter should be in place; and, if possible, another intravenous line should be opened. A purse-string suture of No. 1 silk is placed around the anus to prevent feces escaping during the surgical procedure. The indwelling catheter is taped to the inside of the healthy thigh. In the male, the scrotum is drawn to the sound side and sutured to the inside of the normal thigh above and below the penis. In the female, tamponade of the vagina may be advisable. The patient is placed in side position, with the sound side below.

The skin should be prepared with a bacteriacidal solution from the lower part of the chest to below the knee on the involved side, including the medial aspect of the thigh on the sound side. The unprepared part of the involved leg is dropped into a sterile drape, and the rest of the involved extremity is draped free in such a fashion that the crest of the ileum on that side is accessible all around.

TECHNIQUE

The incision starts at the anterior superior iliac spine, and continues toward the symphysis pubis approximately one finger breadth above the inguinal ligament (Fig. 15-1). The epigastric vessels are ligated and transected (Fig. 15-2). The inguinal canal is entered, and the spermatic cord or round ligament, respectively, is dislocated superiorly with the abdominal muscles. The abdominal wall is now opened, and the peritoneum comes into view. It is retracted medially, exposing the retroperitoneal space. The ureter has to be found, mobilized with a moist sponge, and moved medially with the peritoneal pouch (Fig. 15-3). The common iliac artery is identified, doubly ligated, and divided between the ties. The iliac vein is ligated rather more distally in the region of the external iliac vein. This prevents excessive venous engorgement of the pelvic organs.

The internal iliac artery is then followed into the depths of the pelvis, doubly ligated peripherally to the superior gluteal artery, and then divided.

The posterior part of the skin incision is then made (Fig. 15-4). It follows the iliac crest to the midpoint, turns distally along the greater trochanter, and curves posteriorly and inferiorly following the gluteal fold. On the medial side of the thigh, it follows a line approximately two finger breadths below the ischium. It comes forward anteriorly to cross the insertion of the adductor, and meets the first part of the incision at the symphysis. Since the gluteal muscles remain with the specimen, the interval between the subcutaneous fat and the gluteal fascia has to be developed (Fig. 15-5). This soft tissue flap has to be large enough to expose access to the sacroiliac joint.

Anteriorly, the symphysis pubis is visualized. A curved clamp is passed close to the bone and posteriorly around the pubic bone, and a Gigli saw is drawn through the ensuing canal. The symphysis pubis is then divided (Fig. 15-6). Care must be taken so that no injury is inflicted upon the urethra under the symphysis pubis. On the inside of the pelvis, the psoas muscle is divided at or above the level of the iliac crest. The origin of the quadratus lumborum from the iliac crest is divided. The sacroiliac joint comes into view as the distal stump of the posas muscle is pulled forward. The piriformis muscle is removed from the anterior surface of the sacrum. The roots of the sacral plexus are transected. The sacroiliac joint

can now be enered with a large blade scalpel. Entering the sacroiliac joint can be expedited by spreading the symphysis pubis. The sacrospinous and sacrotuberous ligments, together with muscles of the pelvic floor, are then cut from posterior to anterior. After transecting the posterior attachments of the ilium to the sacrum, the limb can now be removed (Fig. 15-7). The wound is now irrigated, and closure is started by bringing the posterior flap forward and slightly downward. If it is very long, a wedge-shaped section should be removed from the central part. This area lacks blood supply because of the absence of the gluteal artery. The skin must be cut back to a line where fresh bleeding can be observed.[3] A drain is placed into the wound, and the subcutaneous tissue is closed with absorbable sutures. The skin is approximated with interrupted nonabsorbable sutures (Fig. 15-8). The wound is dressed in a bulky dressing.

The patient is kept on a nasogastric tube and intravenous feeding until bowel sounds are established and the patient passes flatus. The drain is advanced; however, the dressing is not changed until approximately five days following the procedure. Ambulation on crutches can be stated 10 to 12 days following the procedure.

A hemipelvectomy can be made more radical by carrying out the posterior transection of the hemipelvis through the wing of the sacrum, rather than the sacroiliac joint.

Figures 15-1 to 15-8.   Hemipelvectomy.

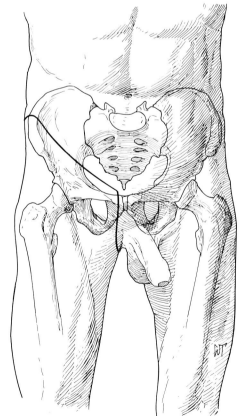

Figure 15-1.   Outline of the anterior part of the skin incision.

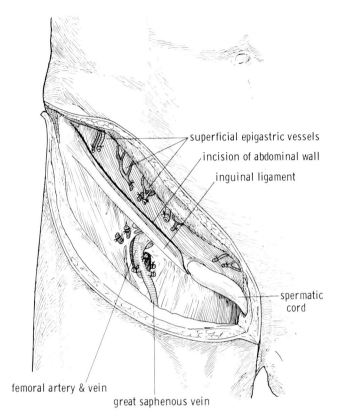

Figure 15-2. Exposure and ligation of the epigastric vessel and the femoral vein and artery.

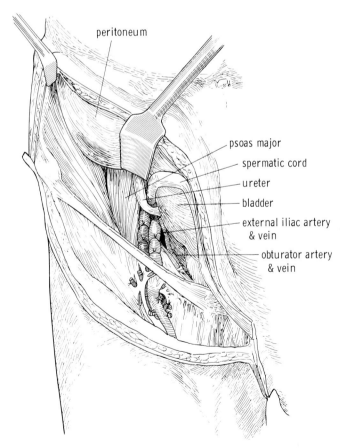

Figure 15-3. Exposure of the abdominal cavity, and ligation of the external iliac vessels.

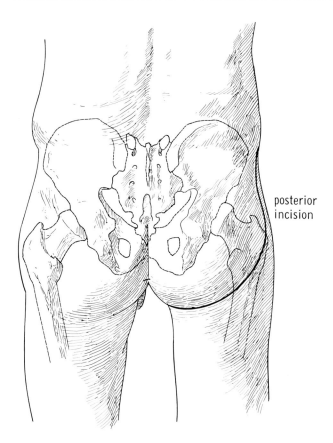

Figure 15-4.   Outline of the posterior part of the incision.

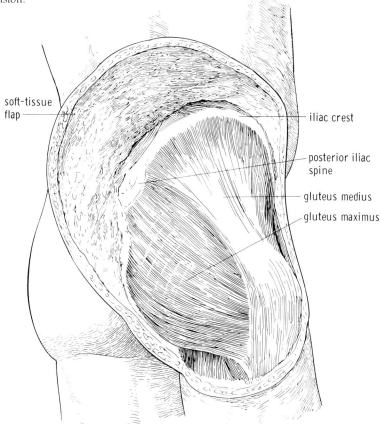

Figure 15-5.   The gluteus maximus and sacroiliac joint area have been exposed.

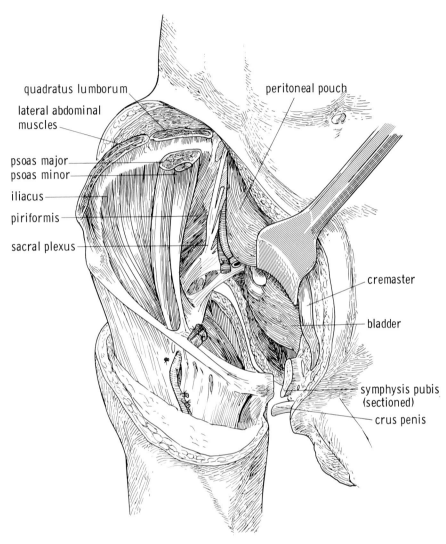

quadratus lumborum

lateral abdominal
muscles

psoas major

psoas minor

iliacus

piriformis

sacral plexus

peritoneal pouch

cremaster

bladder

symphysis pubis
(sectioned)

crus penis

Figure 15-6.   The Symphysis pubis and abdominal muscles have
been transected.

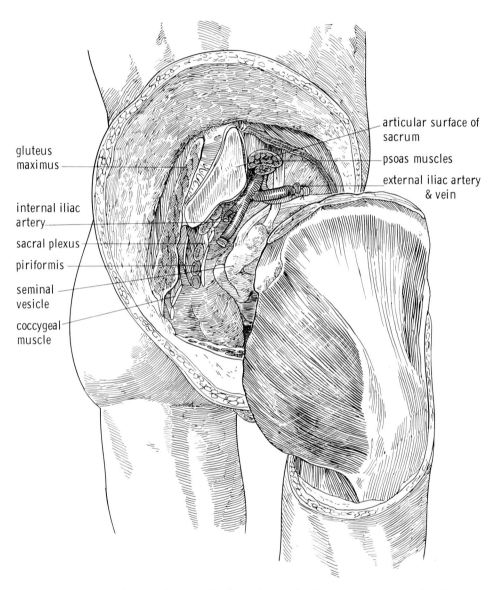

gluteus
maximus

internal iliac
artery

sacral plexus

piriformis

seminal
vesicle

coccygeal
muscle

articular surface of
sacrum

psoas muscles

external iliac artery
& vein

Figure 15-7.   The sacroiliac joint has been disarticulated, amputation is completed.

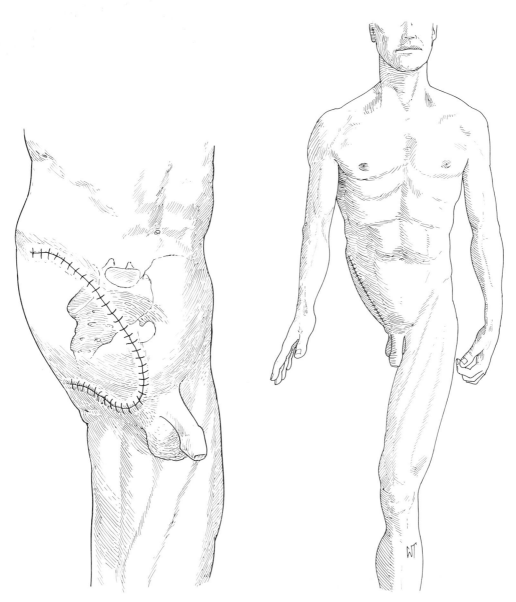

Figure 15-8.   Skin closure.

Technique of Anterior Flap Coverage

The patient is lying on the uninvolved side. The lower extremity of the involved side, the medial side of the uninvolved extremity, and the trunk are prepared and draped. The anus is closed with a purse-string suture, which has to be removed at the end of the procedure. The anterior flap is formed through two incisions, with the first one running from the anterior superior iliac spine to 5 to 10 cm above the knee joint on the lateral side, and the second from the perineum along the adductor musculature to join the first incision (Fig. 15-9). The flap raised in this way contains the anterior thigh musculature and the femoral artery, vein, and nerve (Fig. 15-10). It is folded superiorly and medially, and is covered with moist sponges. The incision follows the iliac crest from the anterior superior iliac spine posteriorly to the midline, and from there inferiorly and very slightly laterally to join the origin of the medial incision. The abdominal muscles are detached from the ileum and the pubic bone. The iliac muscle is raised from the inner table of the ileum and retracted medially (Fig. 15-11). The inguinal ligament is detached from the anterior iliac spine together with the muscle insertions in this region. The pubic bone is freed from all muscle and ligament attachments, and then transected. The ileum is transected immediately laterally from the sacroiliac joint (Figs. 15-9 and 15-11).

By retraction of the iliac muscle medially and of the ileum laterally, the superior and inferior gluteal vessels and sciatic nerve, as well as the obturator nerve and vessels, can be clamped and tied. The psoas and quadratus lumborum muscles in the dorsal part of the wound and pelvic diaphragm inferiorly are transected, and the hemipelvis with the lower extremity can be removed (Fig. 15-12). Further hemostatis is obtained, and large drains are placed into the wounds. The anterior flap is then brought posteriorly and laterally over the defect and, where necessary, trimmed for loose closure (Fig. 15-13).

Figures 15-9 to 15-13.   Modified hemipelvectomy.

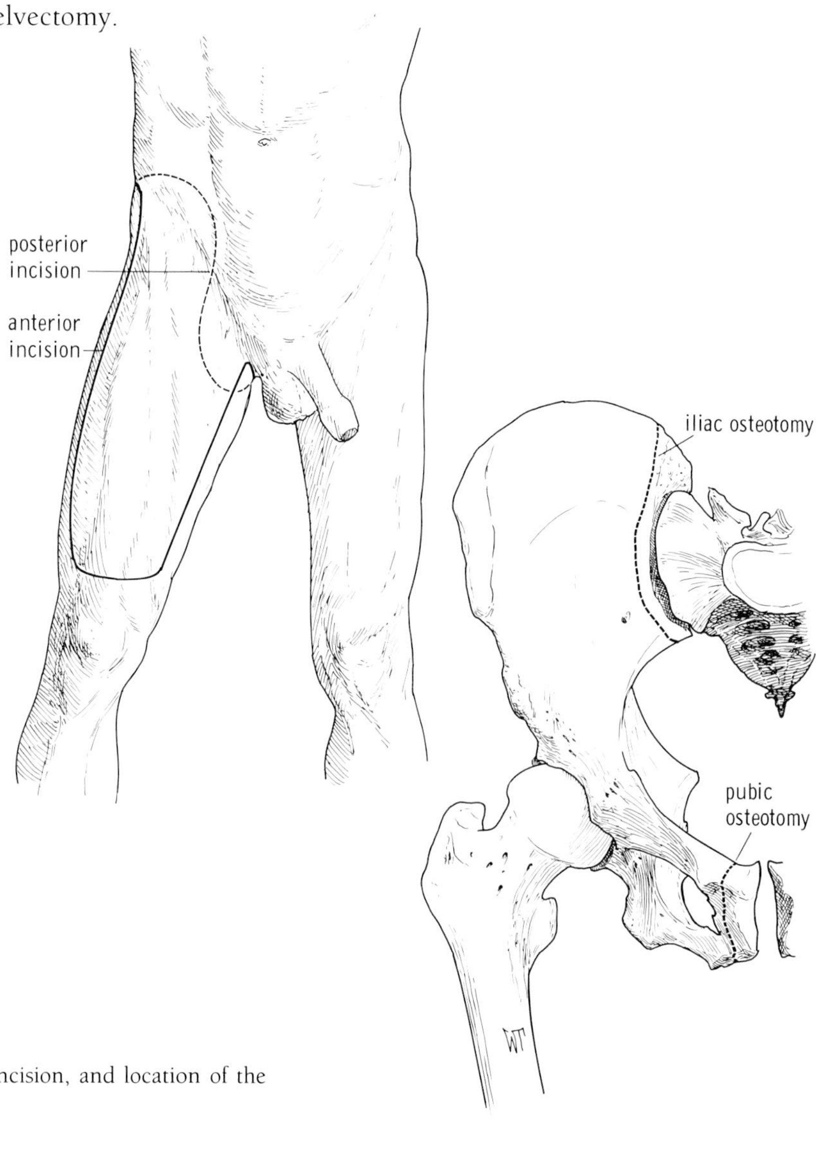

Figure 15-9. Outline of the skin incision, and location of the transection of the pelvic bones.

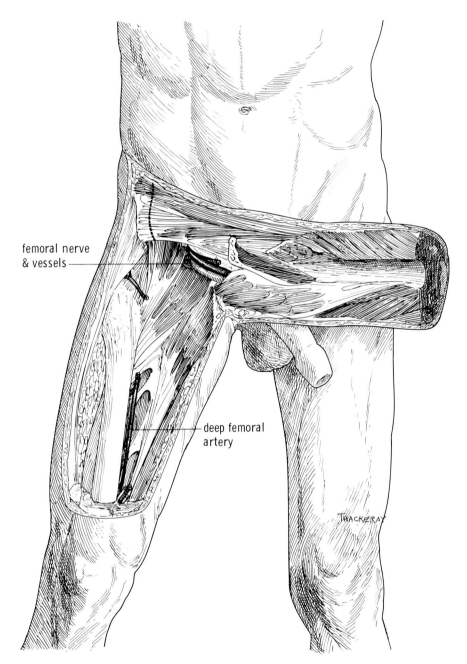

femoral nerve
& vessels

deep femoral
artery

THACKERAY

Figure 15-10.   The anterior thigh flap has been raised.

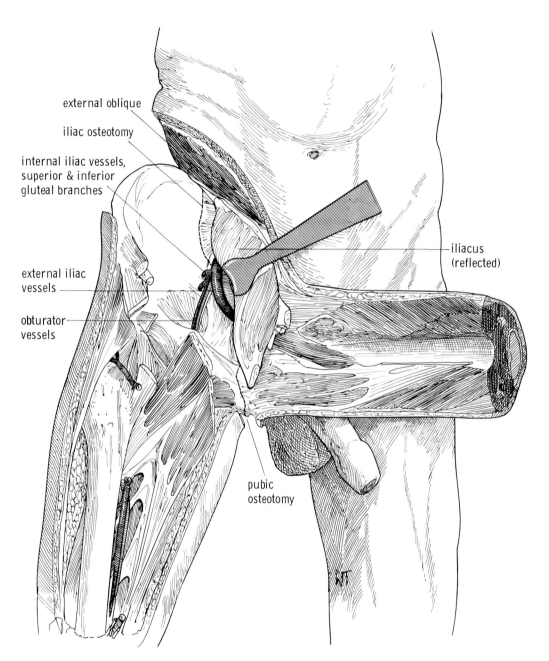

external oblique

iliac osteotomy

internal iliac vessels,
superior & inferior
gluteal branches

external iliac
vessels

obturator
vessels

iliacus
(reflected)

pubic
osteotomy

Figure 15-11.   Exposure of the iliac and gluteal vessels after the iliacus muscle has
been detached from the inner wall of the pelvis.

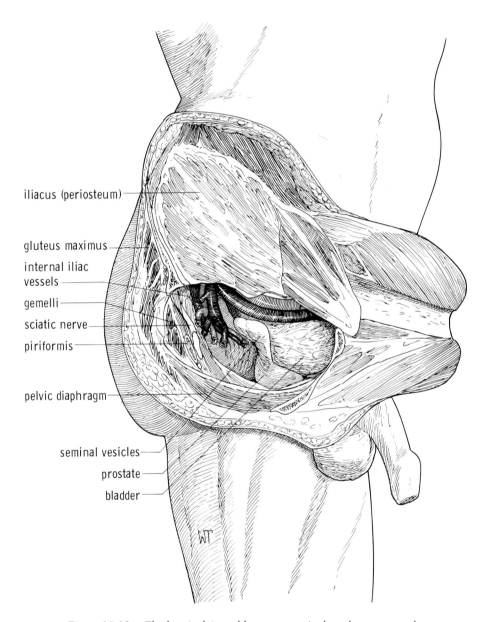

iliacus (periosteum)

gluteus maximus

internal iliac
vessels

gemelli

sciatic nerve

piriformis

pelvic diaphragm

seminal vesicles

prostate

bladder

Figure 15-12.   The hemipelvis and lower extremity have been removed.

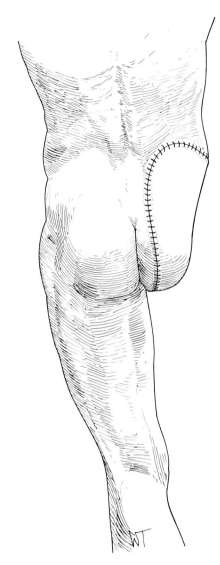

Figure 15-13.   Skin closure.

CONSERVATIVE HEMIPELVECTOMY

In cases where a malignant tumor of the thigh is in the close vicinity of the hip joint, a so-called conservative hemipelvectomy has been described. It is not a hemipelvectomy in the strict sense, as it leaves behind the wing of the ileum attached to the sacroiliac joint. This remaining part of the pelvic skeleton may prove to be an advantage in anchoring the prosthesis. Its disadvantage is loss of the continuity to the opposite part of the hemipelvis and the resultant strain on the sacroiliac joint.[5]

Technique

The patient is in supine position, and the involved side of the hemipelvis is propped up slightly. The incision starts on the sound side of the symphysis pubis, and continues parallel to the inguinal ligament to a point below the anterior superior iliac spine (Fig. 15-14). The incision is continued posteriorly only after the anterior resection has been completed. Skin flaps are raised, and the abdominal muscles are removed from the inguinal ligament (Fig. 15-15). After retraction of the peritoneum medially, the external iliac vessels and the femoral nerve are exposed in the retroperitoneal space (Fig. 15-16). These structures are ligated and transected. Any more proximal lymph nodes can be resected. The iliopsoas muscle is undermined and transected. This exposes the sciatic notch and the adjacent innominate bone (Fig. 15-17). By sharp and blunt dissection, the muscles from the iliac spine are removed, and the gluteus minimus is raised bluntly. A Gigli saw is passed through the sciatic notch, and the innominate bone is transected (Fig. 15-18). After clearing the soft tissue and muscle attachments from around the symphysis pubis, the symphysis is also transected with the Gigli saw.

The skin incision is now continued midway between the tip of the greater trochanter and iliac crest. Posteriorly to the greater trochanter, it continues inferiorly and slightly distal to the gluteal fold into the perineum and ends at the anterior limb of the incision at the symphysis pubis (Fig. 15-19). Skin flaps are raised to expose the gluteus maximus, which is transected (Fig. 15-20). Under it, the gluteus medius and minimus are transected. The gluteal veins and arteries are doubly ligated and transected, and so is the piriformis muscle as well as the sacrotuberous ligament. The sciatic nerve is the last structure to be ligated and transected. Thereafter, the extremity can be removed (Figs. 15-21 and 15-22).

Hemostasis is obtained and the abdominal muscles are sutured to the gluteal muscles with interrupted absorbable sutures (Fig. 15-23). Suction drains are placed into the subcutaneous space, and the skin is closed with interrupted nonabsorbable sutures (Fig. 15-24).

Figures 15-14 to 15-24.   Conservative hemiphelvectomy.

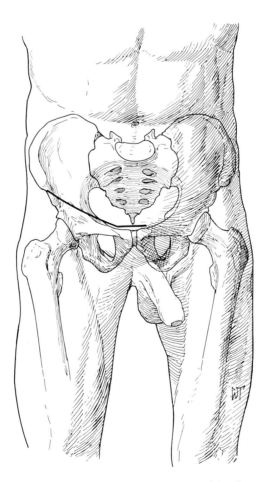

Figure 15-14.   Outline of the anterior part of the skin incision.

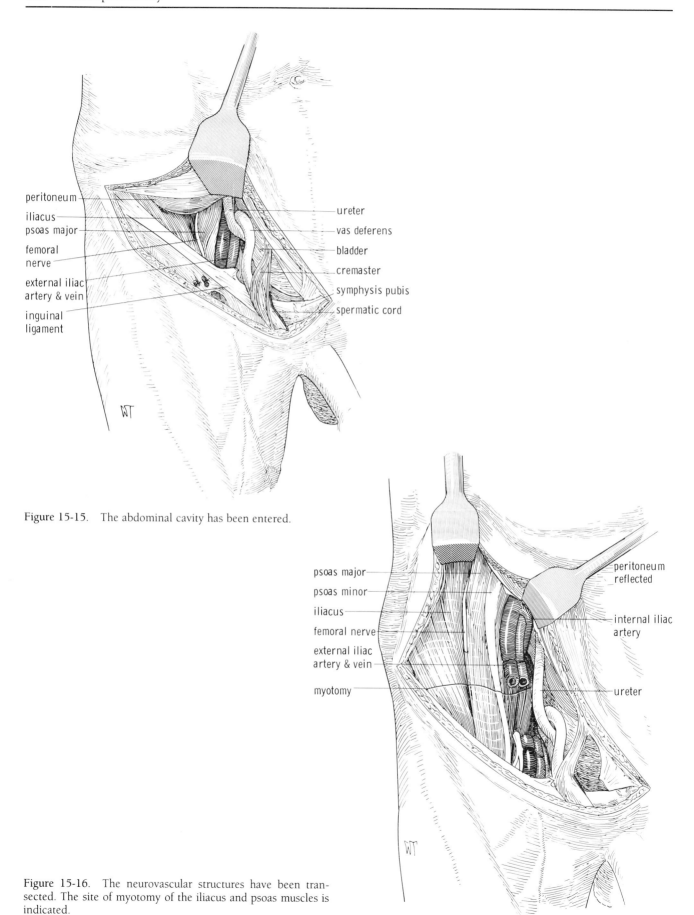

Figure 15-15.   The abdominal cavity has been entered.

Figure 15-16.   The neurovascular structures have been transected. The site of myotomy of the iliacus and psoas muscles is indicated.

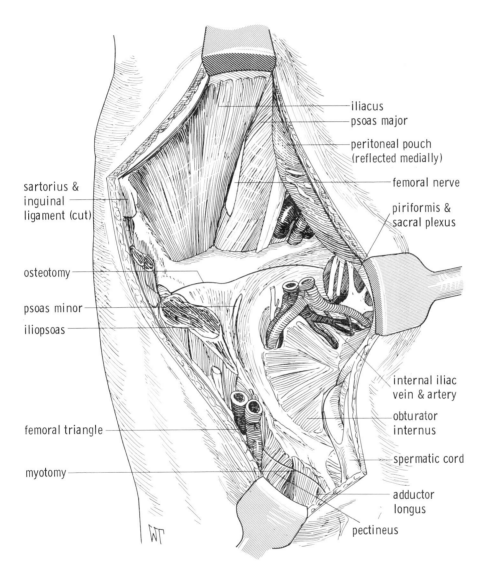

Figure 15-17. The innominate bone has been exposed. The site of the osteotomy is indicated.

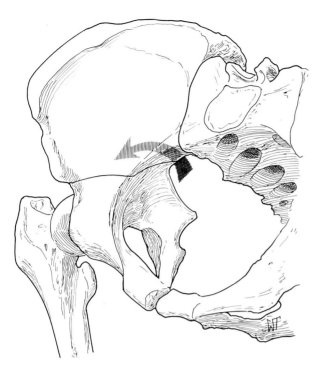

Figure 15-18.   Schematic representation of the site of osteotomy of the innominate bone and symphysis pubis.

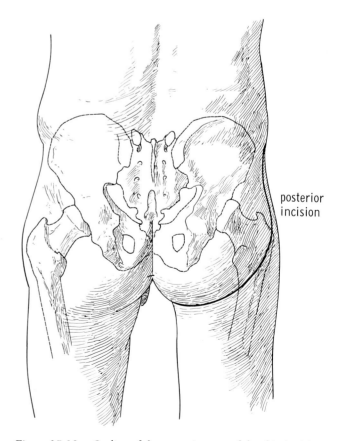

Figure 15-19.   Outline of the posterior part of the skin incision.

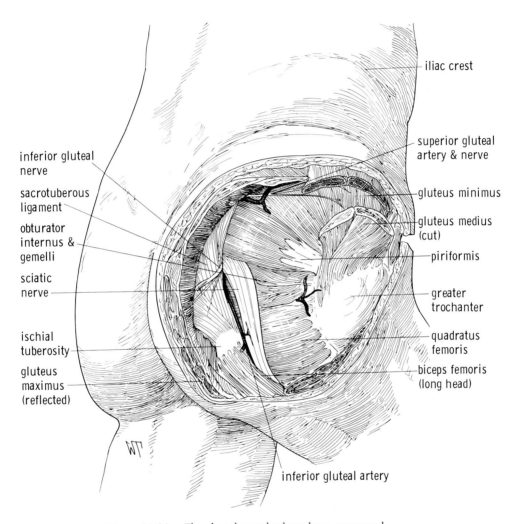

iliac crest

superior gluteal
artery & nerve

inferior gluteal
nerve

gluteus minimus

sacrotuberous
ligament

gluteus medius
(cut)

obturator
internus &
gemelli

piriformis

sciatic
nerve

greater
trochanter

ischial
tuberosity

quadratus
femoris

gluteus
maximus
(reflected)

biceps femoris
(long head)

inferior gluteal artery

Figure 15-20.   The gluteal muscles have been transected.

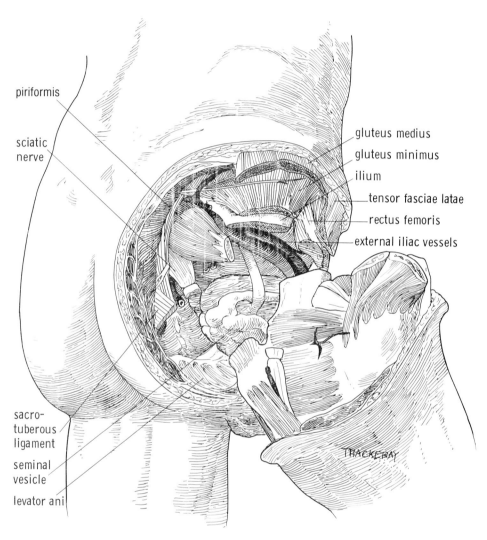

piriformis

sciatic
nerve

gluteus medius

gluteus minimus

ilium

tensor fasciae latae

rectus femoris

external iliac vessels

sacro-
tuberous
ligament

seminal
vesicle

levator ani

THACKERAY

Figure 15-21.   Removal of the inferior part of the pelvis and the lower extremity.

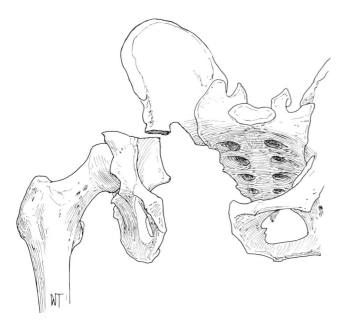

Figure 15-22. Schematic representation of the area of transection of the innominate bone and symphysis pubis.

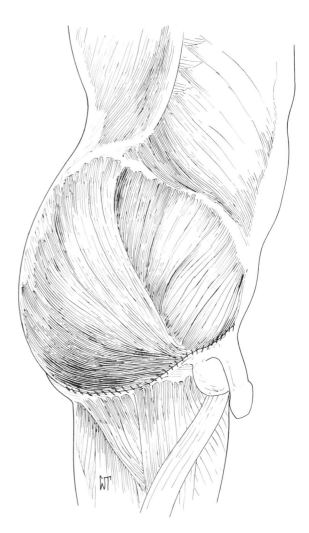

Figure 15-23. Schematic representation of the approximation of the remaining muscles.

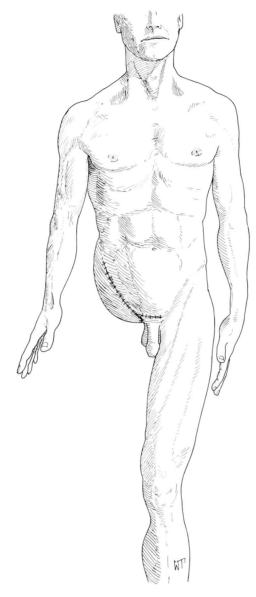

Figure 15-24.   Skin closure.

References

1. Gordon-Taylor G, Monro R: The technique and management of the hindquarter amputation. *Br J Surg* 39:536–541, 1952.

2. Miller TR: Hemipelvectomy in lower extremity tumors. *Orthopaedic Clin North Am* 8:903–919, 1977.

3. Miller TR: 100 cases of hemipelvectomy. A personal experience. *Surg Clin North Am* 54:405–913, 1974.

4. Frey C, Matthews LS, Benjamin H, Fidler WJ: A new technique for hemipelvectomy. *Surg Gynecol Obstet* 143:753–756, 1976.

5. Ariel IM, Shah JP: The conservative hemipelvectomy. *Surg Gynecol Obstet* 144:407–413, 1977.

CHAPTER 16
Finger Amputation

In amputation surgery, the hand occupies a special place. This is mainly due to its triple role. The first function of the hand is that of a prehensile end organ that can deal with the objects within our reach. Its second function is that of a sensory organ. The third function is related to its use as a gesticulating organ, participating in the transmission of information and sometimes supplanting the use of the spoken work —as in with sign language for deaf mutes. These demands on the hands can make the loss of even a small amount of soft tissue a serious mutilation. The prehensile function of the hand exposes it more than any other part of the body to traumatic amputations. The amputating physician should make every effort to save as much of the hand as possible, and make it feasible to render the remnant as close to normal as possible, with good circulation and sensitivity, adequate mobility and dexterity, and adequate strength.[1,2]

MANAGEMENT OF TRAUMATIC FINGERTIP AMPUTATIONS[3]

According to the angle of the denuded surface to the long axis of the phalanx, the fingertip amputations have been divided into three types (Fig. 16-1).[4]

Type I — The denuded surface is perpendicular to the long axis of the phalanx.
Type II — The major part of the denuded surface is on the dorsal aspect of the fingertip.
Type III — The major part of the denuded surface is on the volar aspect.

Depending upon the amount of tissue lost and the surface to be covered, the surgical procedure has to be varied.

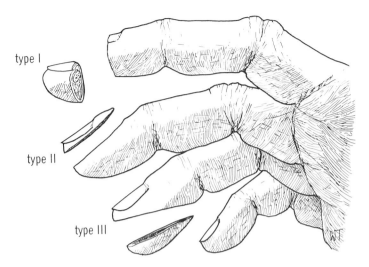

Figure 16-1.   Types of traumatic fingertip amputation.

Type I

The loss of the tip of the pulp lends itself most easily to the Cutler advancement of two lateral flaps that remain attached to the subcutaneous tissue.[5] These flaps are then nourished through the subcutaneous tissue.

Procedure

Under regional or general anesthesia, the extremity is cleansed and draped in the usual fashion (Fig. 16-2). Surgery is undertaken under tourniquet control. The wound is debrided sparingly. Protruding bone spicules are removed. Two equilateral triangular flaps are outlined on the radial and ulnar side of the distal phalanx in such a way that one base coincides with the wound edge, and the proximally pointing apex is in the midlateral line. The base of each triangle should not be more than 4 to 6 mm in length. The skin is then incised, and the subcutane-

ous tissue is mobilized just enough to allow advancement of the flaps toward midline, where the bases are sewn together. The volar part of the defect can then be mobilized as well, and brought up toward the volar part of the two triangular flaps. The ensuing radial and ulnar defect can be closed primarily. The wound is dressed with a sterile bulky dressing after the tourniquet has been released.

A somewhat similar way of coverage of a type I defect is the Atasoy-Kleinert volar VY technique.[6] An equilateral triangle is mapped out on the volar aspect of the distal phalanx, with the base at the cut edge of the skin. This triangle is mobilized in a similar fashion as the flaps in the Cutler procedure. The skin is incised while the subcutaneous tissue remains attached to the underlying bone. The base of the skin triangle is sutured to the remnant of the nail plate, with the sides to the nail wall. The ensuing defect can be closed primarily because of the movement of subcutaneous tissue more distally than the ensuing decrease in bulk.

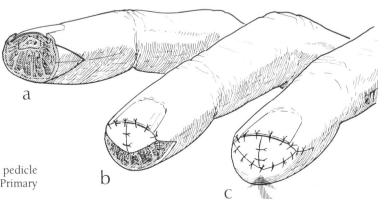

Figure 16-2.   Cutler's advancement. a. Outline of the pedicle flaps. b. Advancement of the flaps toward the midline. c. Primary closure of the remaining defect.

Type II: Bipedicle Dorsal Flap

Where there is an amputation of the fingertip proximally to the nail matrix, the advance of a bipedicle dorsal flap may become advisable.

Technique

After thorough cleansing of the wound and minimal debridement, the skin of the dorsum of the finger is undermined starting at the wound edge and moving proximally (Fig. 16-3). Skin and subcutaneous tissue should be thick enough to leave the areolar tissue covering the extensor apparatus intact. When enough tissue has been raised to cover the original defect, a proximal transverse incision is made. Care has to be taken not to injure the neurovascular bundle. The flap is then brought distally, and its distal edge is sutured to the volar rim of the original defect. The ensuing defect is covered with a split thickness skin graft of approximately 0.4 mm. Both flaps are sutured in place with nonabsorbable suture material.

Where there is too much stress on the flap, the flap can be converted to a unipedical flap, relying for nutrition on only one neurovascular bundle.

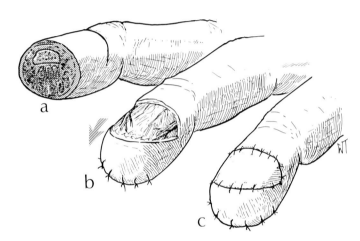

Figure 16-3.   Bipedicle dorsal flap. a. Line of proximal incision. b. Advancement of the flap. c. Split thickness skin coverage of the ensuing defect.

Type III: Volar Bipedicle Flap

In oblique amputations where the volar pulp has been severed, the size of the defect commands the choice of coverage. Amputations of 20 to 30% of the volar surface of the fingertip can be covered by a volar bipedicle flap.[7,8] This flap is obtained through advancement of the volar skin, keeping the radial and ulnar neurovascular bundles intact.

Technique

After cleansing and sparing debridement of the wound, midlateral incisions are made on either side of the digit, starting at the level of the injury and extending to an area proximal to the proximal interphalangeal joint (Fig. 16-4). The neurovascular bundles are identified at this level, and are protected as a transverse incision is made connecting the two midlateral incisions. The entire volar skin and subcutaneous tissue are then mobilized and advanced distally to cover the area of the amputation. Proximal and distal interphalangeal joints have to be flexed slightly to decrease tension on the neurovascular bundles. The flap is then sutured in place with thin, nonabsorbable sutures, starting distally and advancing proximally. After release of the tourniquet, the flexion of the joints of the involved finger may have to be increased to avoid vascular embarrassment of the flap. The finger is put into a splinted dressing, keeping the involved finger in sufficient flexion and also allowing visual access to check the circulation in the flap over the next 48 hours.

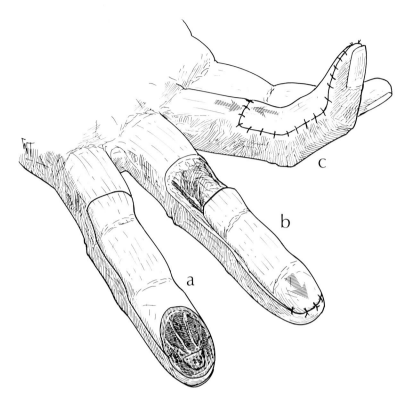

Figure 16-4.   Volar bipedicle flap. a. Outline of the pulp defect. b. Advancement of the volar skin distally. c. Primary closure of the ensuing defect by flexion of the DIP and PIP joints.

Distant Flaps

Where there is surface loss of 50% or more of the distal phalanx, distant flaps may become necessary. These, however, require two surgical procedures: The first procedure requires the raising of the flap and attachment of it to the injured finger; in the second procedure, the flap is detached and set in. Thenar flaps and cross-finger flaps are contraindicated where there are degenerative changes in the finger joints.

Thenar Flap

After sparing debridement and cleansing of the wound, the injured finger is flexed, so that the denuded fingertip touches the thenar eminence and leaves a bloody imprint on it. This blood stain will give the approximate outline of the area of skin to be covered and the location of the skin flap to be raised. The flap itself is raised with its base proximal (Fig. 16-5). Length should be no more than twice its width. The flap must be handled gingerly to avoid tissue

necrosis. The ensuing defects on the thenar eminence and the proximal part of the raw surface of the flap are covered with a thick split thickness graft (Fig. 16-6). The distal edge of the flap is then sutured to the dorsal edge of the wound at the fingertip. It may become necessary to pass sutures through the edge of the nail. The medial and lateral edges of the flap are sutured to the corresponding areas at the finger tip. The thenar flap must not fold back on itself, thereby obstructing the nutrient vessels. Wet cotton is placed over the split thickness graft, and a bulky dressing is applied to the hand, keeping the finger in proper position. It is advisable to leave the graft exposed to check its circulation.

The second procedure—the detachment of the flap—follows two to three weeks after the first. At that time, the base of the thenar flap is detached and set into the proximal edge of the wound at the fingertip. The split thickness graft at the thenar eminence is sutured to the former base of the flap (Fig. 16-7).

Melone et al. recommend as the donor site the area near the metacarpophalangeal joint crease of the thumb. This area provides sufficient bulk for the pulp of the finger, and decreases the risk of stiffness in the proximal interphalangeal joint of the recipient finger.[9]

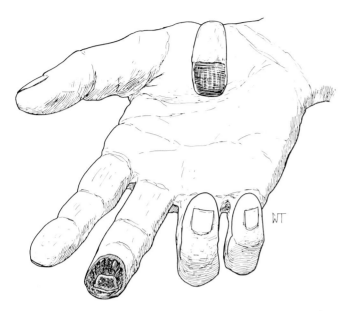

Figure 16-5. Thenar flap. The flap has been raised and is ready to be attached to the defect.

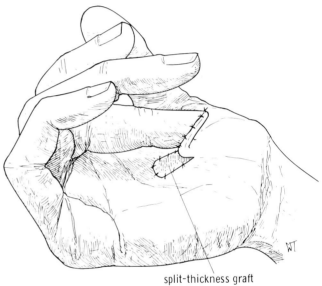

split-thickness graft

Figure 16-6. The thenar flap has been attached, and the ensuing defect covered with a split thickness graft.

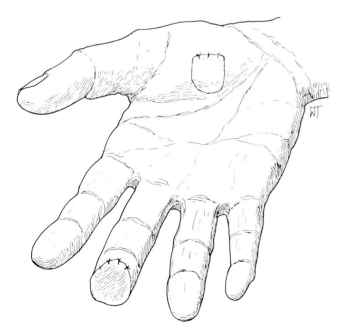

Figure 16-7. The thenar flap has been detached, and the edges of the full thickness as well as the split thickness graft have been set in.

Cross-Finger Flap

The finger tip is prepared in such a way that the defect becomes more or less rectangular (Fig. 16-8). The dimensions of the defect are measured and outlined on the dorsum of the neighboring finger. The flap itself should be 2 to 3 mm wider than the injured surface. The flap is now raised from the dorsum of the donor finger in such a way that the base remains on the side of the recipient finger. It should not cross the midlateral line of the donor finger. The flap is raised with the subcutaneous tissue; however, the peritenon covering the extensor apparatus must be left in place. The donor area is covered with a thick split thickness graft. The pedicle flap is then attached so that the entire recipient area is covered by the graft. The free edge of the split thickness graft can be sutured to the adjacent area of the injury.

A bulky dressing is applied, keeping the fingers in the position that allows good perfusion of the pedicle graft. Part of the graft should be left exposed to allow observation of its blood supply.

The second procedure for detachment of the graft follows after two weeks. The detached margin of the graft is set into the defect, and the free margin of the split thickness graft is used to fully cover the donor site. Early active motion of the fingers is necessary to ensure restoration of mobility.

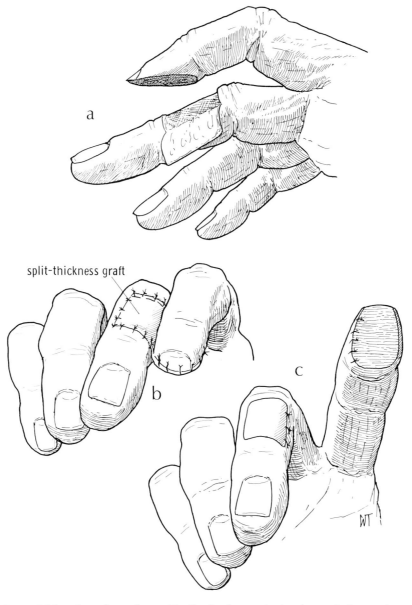

split-thickness graft

Figure 16-8. Cross-finger flap. a. The flap has been raised and is ready for attachment. b. The pedicle flap has been attached, and the defect is covered with a split thickness graft. c. The pedicle flap has been detached, and the pedicle as well as the split thickness grafts have been set in.

PLANNING OF FINGER AMPUTATIONS[10]

In the planning of amputations of the fingers, it must be kept in mind that each finger maintains a unique position among its neighbors and fulfills a special function. The surgeon should strive for the maintenance of as much length as possible. One should keep in mind not only maintenance of the length of the fingers, but also the width of the palm. In a secondary procedure, ray resection and transposition of rays become necessary. Where disarticulation is advisable to maintain the length, the joint cartilage should be preserved,[11] and only the volar condyle and the medial and lateral flare of the phalanx should be removed. If at all possible, the scar should be placed toward the dorsal aspect of the finger.

Levels of Amputation[12]

Thumb

Since the thumb is the only opposable digit, it is of more value than any other finger. Even a small amount of loss in length can represent a serious handicap. After loss of the entire thumb through the metacarpophalangeal joint, an opposable post may be gained by deepening the first web space and phalangizing the first metacarpal.

Index Finger[13,14]

It provides the second branch in the pinch grasp with the thumb. Thus, when the distal end of the index finger is lost, this ability to prehension is also lost, and it has to be transferred to the middle finger. This often decreases dexterity considerably. However, the index finger also provides, together with the middle finger, a strong grasp in holding large objects. Thus, maintenance of the middle and proximal phalanx may become advisable. Certainly in multiple finger amputations, even relatively small stumps of the proximal phalanx are of great help. However, in a single-finger amputation proximal to the head of the proximal phalanx, the stump very often gets into the way; thus, in a second surgical procedure, resection of the first ray may have to be carried out. This will widen the first web space and strengthen the pinch grip with the middle finger.

Middle Finger

Its value is almost similar to that of the next finger. The strength it lends to the hand in grasping and holding onto large objects is equal to that of the index finger. Loss of more than half of the middle phalanx decreases the ability of the hand to form an effective cup, and small objects fall out of the clenched fist. If there is loss of part or all of the metacarpal of the middle finger, the metacarpal row becomes unstable because of the absence of the uniting transverse metacarpal ligament. The central matacarpal also provides the origin for the adductor pollicis muscle. Thus, with amputations through the middle phalanx and certainly after amputations through the third metacarpal, serious consideration should be given to transposition of the second metacarpal upon the base of the third.[15–17]

Ring Finger

Together with the little finger, the ring finger provides mobility of the ulnar side of the hand. Because of this greater mobility, it may be possible for the patient to form an effective cup with the hand, even after loss of the fingers through the proximal interphalangeal joint. However, after amputations proximal to that point, consideration should be given to resection of the remaining part of the fourth ray through the base of the fourth metacarpal, and to transposition of the fifth upon the fourth metacarpal.[17,18]

Little Finger

In single-finger amputations, loss of the fifth finger is the least disconcerting for the patient. The cosmetic appearance of the hand can often be improved upon by a secondary resection of the metacarpal, which should be done obliquely at the base to avoid protrudences.

TECHNIQUE OF FINGER AMPUTATION

After adequate preparation and under tourniquet control, skin flaps are outlined (Fig. 16-9). Where possible, the volar flap should be longer so that it covers the ensuing tip of the stump. The incision is carried through the skin and subcutaneous tissue, and neurovascular bundles are exposed. Arteries and veins are ligated separately. The digital nerves are dissected free to a point well proximal to the level of bony transection and cut. The flexor tendon sheath is entered. Since each phalanx has its own flexor mechanism, the flexor tendon to the more distal phalanx can be pulled out of the tendon sheath and transected. After release of the tourniquet, further hemostasis is obtained, and the skin is closed with thin, nonabsorbable sutures. A bulky dressing is applied.

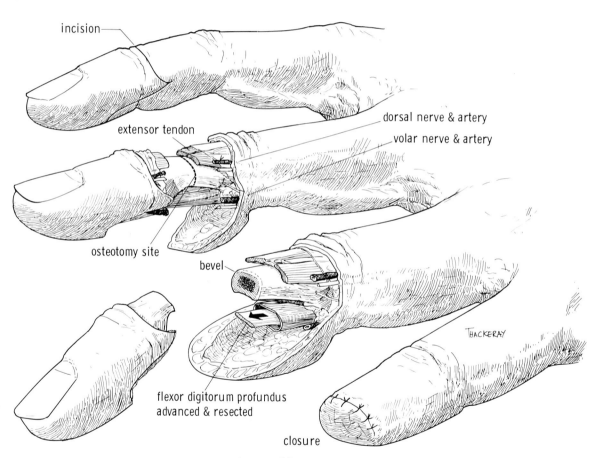

Figure 16-9.   Technique of finger amputation.

TECHNIQUE OF FINGER DISARTICULATION

The level of the finger joint to be disarticulated is determined (Fig. 16-10). After adequate preparation and under tourniquet control, the skin flaps are outlined, leaving the volar flap longer than the dorsal flap. The incision is carried through the subcutaneous tissue along the outline. The neurovascular bundles are identified, veins and arteries ligated, and the digital nerves are resected well proximal to the level of the disarticulation. The collateral ligaments of the finger joint are dissected, the capsule is opened, and the disarticulation is completed in this way. The transected tendons are pulled into the wound and cut off so they can retract. The joint cartilage is left intact.[11] The volar condyle of the remaining phalanx may need to be trimmed. The tourniquet is released, hemostases are obtained, and the skin is closed with nonabsorbable sutures, keeping the scar on the dorsal aspect of the stump.

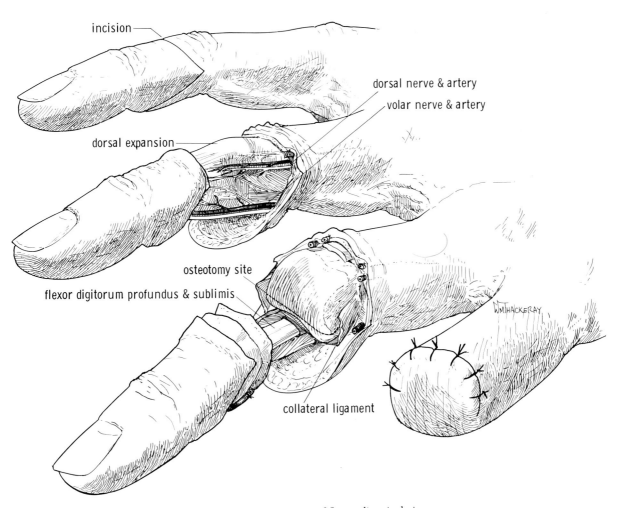

Figure 16-10.   Technique of finger disarticulation.

Disarticulation of the Thumb and Deepening of the First Web Space[17]

After adequate preparation and inflation of the tourniquet, the skin incision is outlined, including the preparation of Z-plasty in the first web space (Fig. 16-11). After the thumb has been disarticulated at the proximal interphalangeal joint, the flaps of the Z-plasty are raised in such a way that the volar flap is used to ultimately cover the thenar post. The first dorsal interosseus muscle is teased off its origin from the first metacarpal extraperiosteally. The insertion of the adductor pollicis is transferred to a more proximal position in the first metacarpal (Fig. 16-12). Skin closure is then obtained by advancement of the dorsal and volar flaps of the Z-plasty (Fig. 16-13). A short but usually quite powerful thumb post is gained (Fig. 16-14).

Figures 16-11 to 16-14.   Thumb disarticulation and deepening of the first web space.

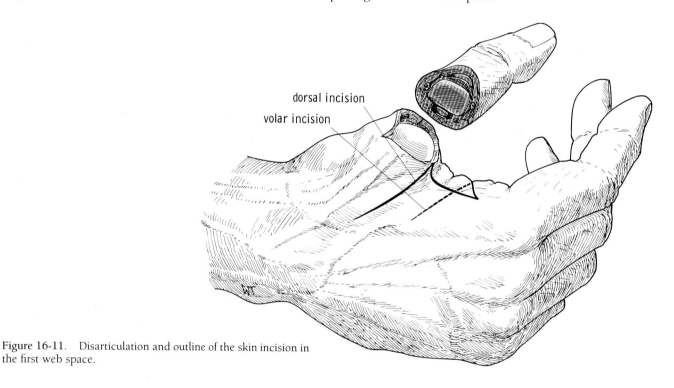

Figure 16-11.   Disarticulation and outline of the skin incision in the first web space.

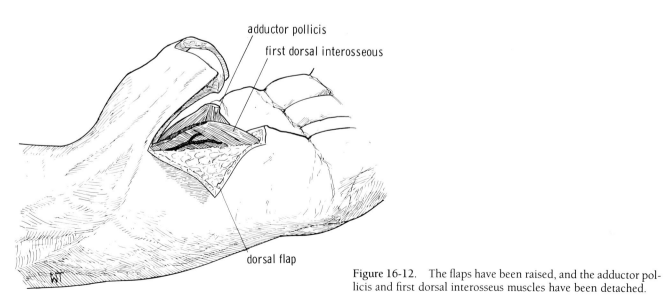

Figure 16-12.   The flaps have been raised, and the adductor pollicis and first dorsal interosseus muscles have been detached.

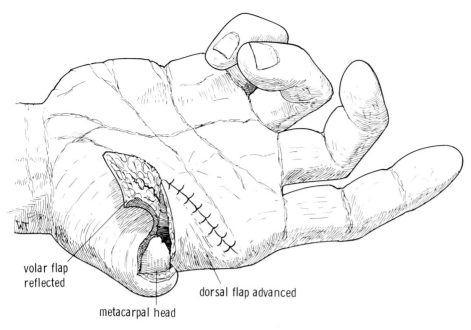

volar flap
reflected

metacarpal head

dorsal flap advanced

Figure 16-13.   First step in the closure.

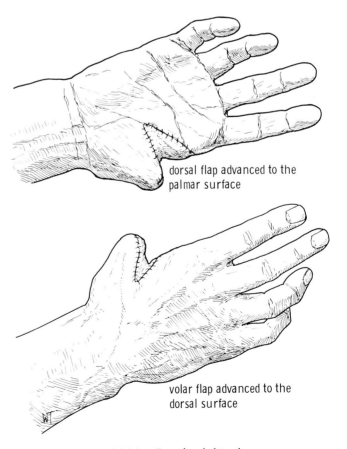

dorsal flap advanced to the
palmar surface

volar flap advanced to the
dorsal surface

Figure 16-14.   Completed skin closure.

METACARPAL AMPUTATION

Where there is a primary amputation through the metacarpal and no immediate transposition of the adjacent metacarpal is contemplated, enough of the proximal end of the metacarpal should be kept in place to allow for transposition of the metacarpal at a later date. Also, the amount of skin resected from the volar and dorsal aspects of the hand should be sparing. Tight closures can lead to skin sloughs at the height of posteroperative swelling.

Technique

After adequate preparation and inflation of the tourniquet, the incisions are outlined. After incision of the skin and the subcutaneous tissue, the common digital artery is exposed. Where at all possible, only the proper digital arteries to the finger to be amputated should be ligated and transected. The digital nerves are transected as far proximally as possible by splitting their respective common digital nerve.

First Metacarpal

As much of the proximal end of the metacarpal should be preserved to facilitate deepening of the first web space or transposition of the index finger at a later date in an attempt to pollicisize that index finger (Figs. 16-15 and 16-16). Resection of the bone should be done subperiosteally to maintain as much of the thenar musculature as possible.

Figures 16-15 and 16-16.   Pollicization.

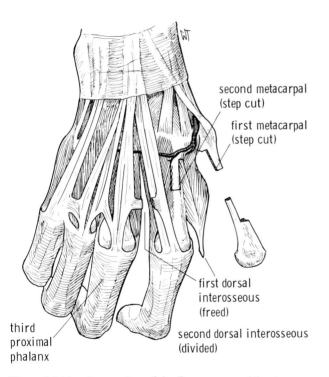

Figure 16-15.   Preparation of the first metacarpal for the transposition.

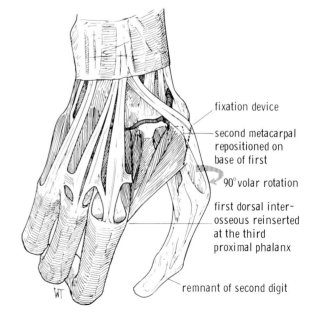

Figure 16-16.   Completed pollicization.

Second Metacarpal[13]

The first dorsal interosseous muscle is carefully detached from the insertion on the radial aspect of the proximal phalanx. The metacarpal is resected close to its base, if at all possible, distally to the insertion of the extensor carpi radialis longus. Through a drill hole in the base of the proximal phalanx of the middle finger, the tendon of the first dorsal interosseous is reattached to the middle finger by means of a pull-out suture. The tourniquet is released and hemostasis is obtained. The wound is closed with thin, nonabsorbable sutures.

Third Metacarpal

Care should be taken to maintain enough of the base of the metacarpal so that later transposition of the second upon the third metacarpal is possible. After resection of the metacarpal, the second dorsal interosseous muscle is removed as well. The origin of the adductor muscle of the thumb has to be reattached into the shaft of the fourth metacarpal.

Fourth Metacarpal

Sufficient length has to be maintained to allow later transposition of the fifth metacarpal upon the fourth metacarpal.

Fifth Metacarpal

An attempt should be made to preserve the abductor digiti quinti muscle and insert it into the base of the proximal phalanx of the ring finger. The resection at the base of the fifth metacarpal should be oblique to avoid any unsightly projections. It is not advisable to retain any part of the shaft of the fifth metacarpal.

References

1. Steinbach T-V: Upper limb amputation. *Prog Surg* 16:224–248, 1978.
2. Wilson RL, Carter-Wilson M: Rehabilitation after amputations in the hand. *Orthopaedic Clin North Am* 14(4):851–872, 1983.
3. Rosenthal EA: Treatment of fingertip and nail bed injuries. Orthopaedic Clin North Am 14(4):675–697, 1983.
4. Sokol AB, Berggren RB: Finger tip amputations— Review of procedures and applications. *Calif Med* 119:22–28, 1973.
5. Glicenstein J: Les amputation des extremites digitales. *Acta Orthopaedica Belgica* 39:1148–1156, 1973.
6. Atasoy E, Ioakimidis E, Kasdan ML, et al: Reconstruction of the amputated finger tip with a triangular volar flap. A new surgical procedure. *J Bone Joint Surg* 52A:921–926, 1970.
7. Millender LH, Albin RE, Nalebuff EA: Delayed volar advancement flap for thumb tip injuries. *Plastic Reconstr Surg* 52:635–639, 1973.
8. Snow JW: The use of a volar flap for repair of fingertip amputations: A preliminary report. *Plastic Reconstr Surg* 40:163–168, 1967.
9. Melone CP, Beasley RW, Carstens JH: The thenar flap —Analysis of its use in 150 cases. *J Hand Surg* 7:291–297, 1982.
10. Swanson AB: Levels of amputation of fingers and hand —Consideration for treatment. *Surg Clin North Am* 44-4:1115–1126, 1964.
11. Whitaker LA, Graham WP, Riser WH, Kilgore E: Retaining the articular cartilage in finger joint amputations. *Plastic and Reconstr Surg* 19:542–547, 1972.
12. Alnot JY, Duparc J, May P: Amputations uni-digitales des doigts. *Acta Orthopaedica Belgica* 39:1135–1147, 1973.
13. Jandeaux M, Kanhouche R: L'amputation de l'index selon Chase. *Acta Orthopaedica Belgica* 39:1162–1169, 1973.
14. Murray JF, Carman W, MacKenzie JK: Transmetacarpal amputation of the index finger: A clinical assessment of handstrength and complications. *J Hand Surg* 2:471–481, 1977.
15. Posner MA: Ray transposition for central digital loss. *J Hand Surg* 4:242–257, 1979.
16. Razemon JP: La transposition de l'index sur le troisieme metacarpien dans les sequelles d'amputation du medius. *Acta Orthopaedica Belgica* 39:1170–1174, 1973.
17. Tubiana R, Roux J-P: Phalangization of the first and fifth metacarpals. *J Bone Joint Surg* 56-A:447–457, 1974.
18. Rinaldi E, Lacovara V: La transplantation de l'index ou de l'auriculaire dans les sequelles d'amputation d'un doigt central. *Acta Orthopaedica Belgica* 39:1175–1178, 1973.

CHAPTER 17

Carpo-Metacarpal and Transcarpal Amputation and Wrist Disarticulation

CARPO-METACARPAL AND TRANSCARPAL AMPUTATION

The aim of the preservation of either all or a portion of the carpus is to provide an end organ with some flexion and extension, and to maintain palmar skin with its tactile characteristics as well as its ability to pronate and supinate. Sufficient palmar skin with normal neurovascular conditions must be available. Adequate range of motion must be present in the radiocarpal joint and the distal radioulnar joint.

Technique

The arm is prepared and draped, and the tourniquet is inflated. The level of amputation is determined by the skin available for coverage and, of course, by the disease leading to amputation. The lateral apex of the skin incision for a transcarpal amputation lies slightly dorsal to the tip of the radial styloid, with the medial apex slightly ventral to the ulnar styloid. The dorsal flap extends to the carpo-metacarpal joints in a shallow arc, and the palmar incision extends over the thenar eminence to the proximal palmar crease on the radial side and the distal palmar crease on the ulnar side of the palm. For the carpo-metacarpal amputation, the line of incision is placed approximately 2 cm further distally. (Figure 17-1 illustrates both incisions.) The two flaps are then raised sufficiently to expose the level of the transection of the bone (Figs. 17-2 and 17-5). The tendons of the extrinsic

muscles to the fingers are then pulled into the wound and cut short enough to enable them to retract to a level proximal to the wrist joint (Figs. 17-3, 17-4, and 17-6). Care has to be taken to identify the flexors and extensors of the wrist. If the level of amputation is proximal to their insertion, they should be tagged with nonabsorbable sutures and reinserted into the remaining part of the carpus after amputation.

Of the nerves, the median nerve is most easily found in the carpal tunnel. It is dissected up into the forearm and transected well away from the level of the amputation, but distal to the origin of the palmar branch. The ulnar nerve in Guion's canal and its superficial branch are treated in the same fashion (Fig. 17-3). Care has to be taken to find and dissect out the branches of the superficial radial nerve on the dorso-radial aspect of the wrist, as these can lead to painful neuromas.

The carpo-metacarpal or intercarpal joint, as the procedure indicates, is then entered, the amputation is completed, and the bony prominences are smoothed over (Figs. 17-7 to 17-10). The radial artery, ulnar artery, and as many of the dorsal veins as can be seen while the tourniquet is inflated are ligated above the level of the amputation. The tourniquet is then deflated, hemostasis is obtained, and the flexor and extensor tendons of the wrist are then sutured into the ligaments of the carpus where necessary (Figs. 17-11 and 17-12). A suction drain is inserted into the wound; the skin is closed by loose approximation. Figure 17-13 illustrates the final appearance.

146

Figures 17-1 to 17-13.   Carpo-metacarpal and transcarpal amputation.

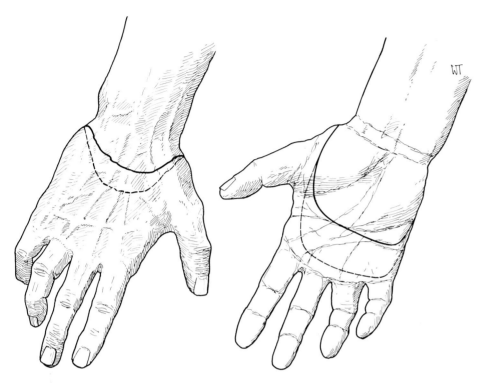

Figure 17-1.   Outline of the incision. The broken line indicates the incision for the carpometacarpal amputation; the solid line indicates the incision for the transcarpal amputation.

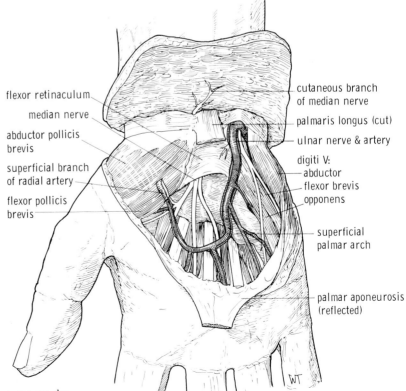

Figure 17-2.   Exposure of the subcutaneous structures on the volar aspect and transection of the palmeris longus.

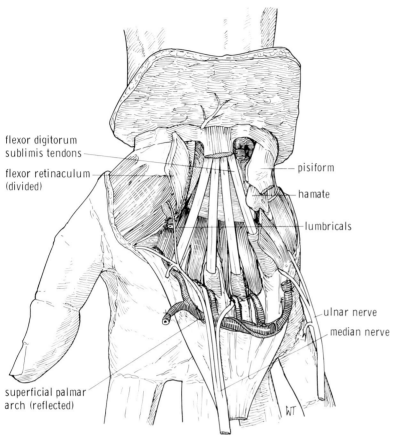

flexor digitorum
sublimis tendons

flexor retinaculum
(divided)

pisiform

hamate

lumbricals

ulnar nerve

median nerve

superficial palmar
arch (reflected)

Figure 17-3.   The flexor digitorum sublimis has been exposed
after transection of the median and ulnar nerves.

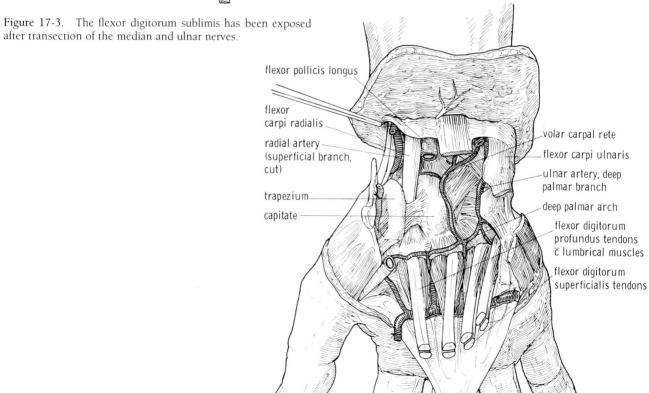

flexor pollicis longus

flexor
carpi radialis

radial artery
(superficial branch,
cut)

trapezium

capitate

volar carpal rete

flexor carpi ulnaris

ulnar artery, deep
palmar branch

deep palmar arch

flexor digitorum
profundus tendons
c̄ lumbrical muscles

flexor digitorum
superficialis tendons

Figure 17-4.   Extrinsic flexor tendons to the fingers have been
transected and turned down distally.

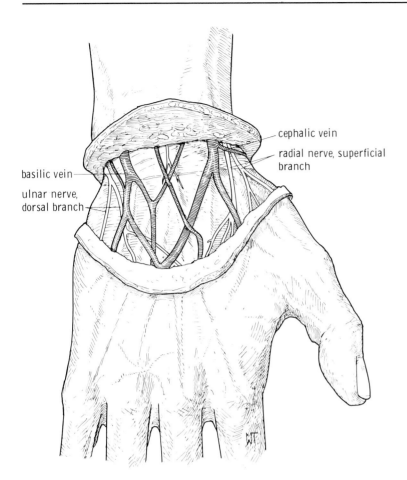

cephalic vein

radial nerve, superficial branch

basilic vein

ulnar nerve, dorsal branch

Figure 17-5. Exposure of the subcutaneous structures on the dorsal aspect of the wrist.

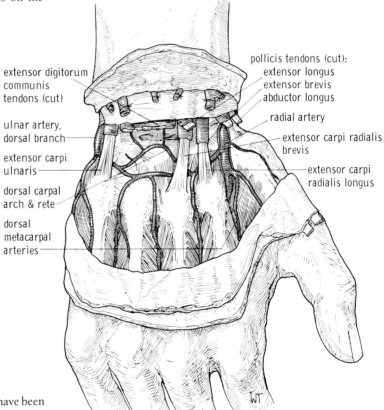

extensor digitorum communis tendons (cut)

pollicis tendons (cut):
extensor longus
extensor brevis
abductor longus

ulnar artery, dorsal branch

radial artery

extensor carpi ulnaris

extensor carpi radialis brevis

dorsal carpal arch & rete

extensor carpi radialis longus

dorsal metacarpal arteries

Figure 17-6. Extrinsic extensor tendons to the fingers have been transected.

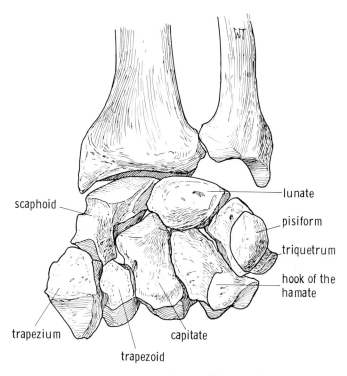

Figure 17-7.   Anatomic relation of the carpal bones.

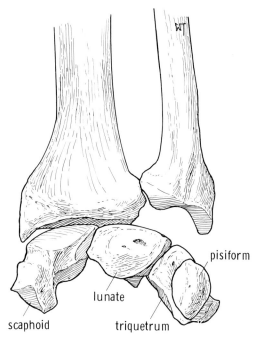

Figure 17-8.   Anatomic relation of the carpal bones.

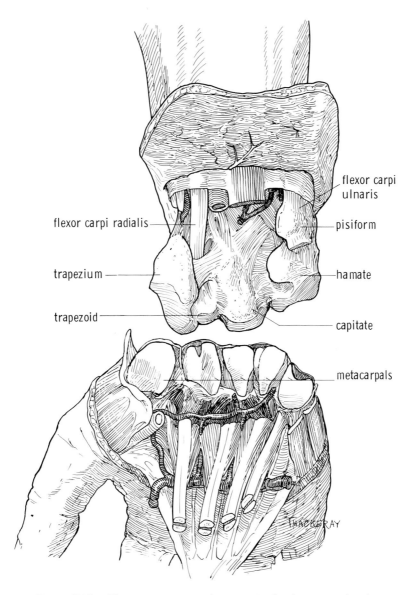

flexor carpi ulnaris

flexor carpi radialis

pisiform

trapezium

hamate

trapezoid

capitate

metacarpals

THACKERAY

Figure 17-9. The carpo-metacarpal amputation has been completed.

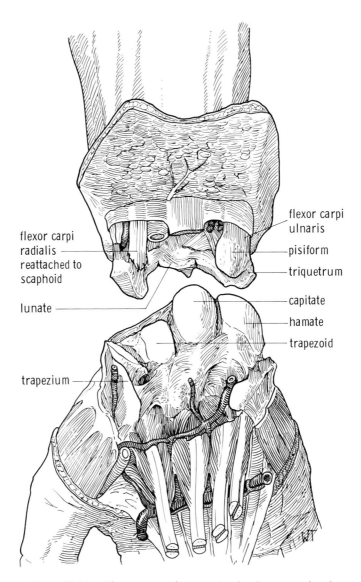

Figure 17-10.   The transcarpal amputation has been completed.

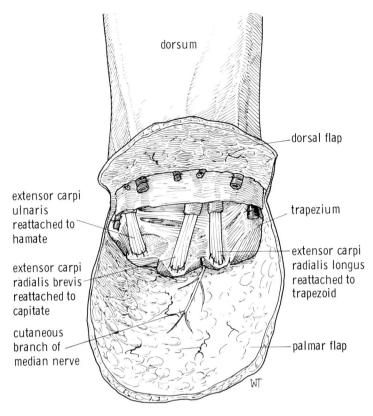

Figure 17-11.   The wrist extensor tendons have been sutured in place in case of the carpo-metacarpal amputation.

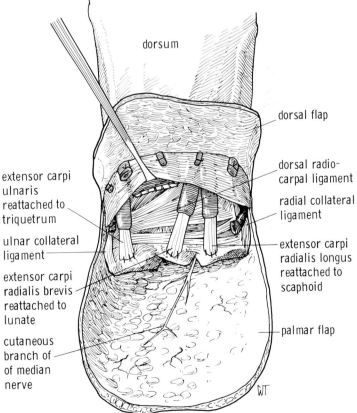

Figure 17-12.   The wrist extensor tendons have been secured to the carpal ligaments in the case of transcarpal amputation.

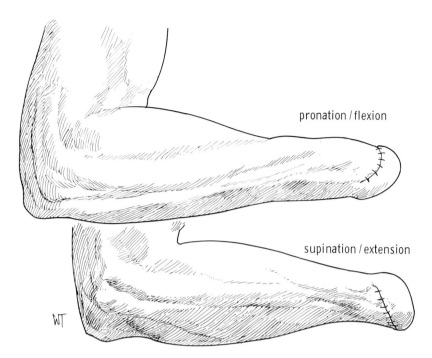

pronation / flexion

supination / extension

Figure 17-13.   Positioning of the skin suture in pronation and flexion and supination and extension, respectively.

WRIST DISARTICULATION

The aim of this procedure is to create an oval-shaped or somewhat rectangular stump. The scar should remain slightly posterior to the line between the tips of the styloid processes. The distal radiocarpal joint must be maintained, and the triangular fibro-cartilage complex should be preserved.

Technique

The extremity is prepared and draped, and the tourniquet is inflated. The skin incision starts at the bottom of the anatomic snuff box, follows a gently curved line distally toward the volar aspect of the first carpo-metacarpal joint, and continues through the heel of the hand in such a fashion that approximately 3 cm of palmar skin are preserved. At the volar aspect of the fifth carpo-metacarpal joint, the incision curves up toward the midmedial line to the level of the hamate. The dorsal part of the incision lies over the proximal carpal row (Fig. 17-14). After reflecting the skin with the subcutaneous tissue, the radial and ulnar arteries are exposed (Fig. 17-15), ligated, and transected. The median and ulnar nerves are identified, followed up into the forearm, and transected (Fig. 17-16). The radial nerve is more difficult to find in the subcutaneous tissue of the radiodorsal aspect of the wrist (Fig. 17-17). The radial aspect of the naviculoradial joint is now identified (Fig. 17-18), and the joint is opened. By extension and ulnar adduction, the dissection is carried on through the tendons on the dorsal and volar aspect of the wrist (Figs. 17-19 and 17-20). These tendons are transected after they have been pulled into view. Great care has to be taken to preserve the triradiate cartilage and the underlying radioulnar joint. The hand is thus amputated. The tourniquet is then deflated, hemostasis is obtained, and the skin is closed over the drain (Fig. 17-21).

It is interesting to note that it is not always necessary to trim the styloid processes, although they have to be resected if they are uncomfortably protrudent. Similarly, the joint cartilage from the radius and the ulna does not have to be removed.

Since the skin of the palm is usually well vascularized, atypical flaps can easily be fashioned. The best known flaps are the thenar and hypothenar flaps.

The thenar flap is fashioned by starting the incision at the depth of the anatomic snuff box. It encircles the volar skin of the entire thenar eminence and part of the first web space. The distal extent is at the metacarpophalangeal joint of the thumb. The ulnar limb of the incision aims to the ulnar side of the first carpo-metacarpal joint. The amount of dorsal skin depends upon the injury and the amount of skin present. After the amputation, the thenar flap is swung toward the ulna in such a fashion that the skin from the metacarpophalangeal joint covers the area of the ulnar styloid.

The hypothenar flap is fashioned by starting the radial incision over the ulnar aspect of the first carpo-metacarpal joint, continuing through the palm toward the fifth metacarpophalangeal joint and proximally over the ulnar border of the fifth metacarpal.

In both flaps, skin and muscles are preserved and an attempt is made to save the innervation of those muscles.

Stumps covered with skin from the dorsum of the hand require either reamputation or conversion into a Krukenberg plasty.

Figures 17-14 to 17-21.   Wrist disarticulation.

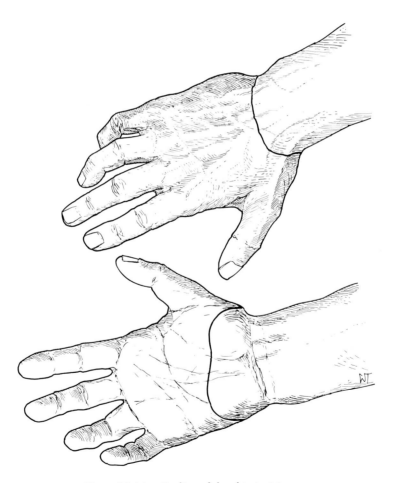

Figure 17-14.   Outline of the skin incision.

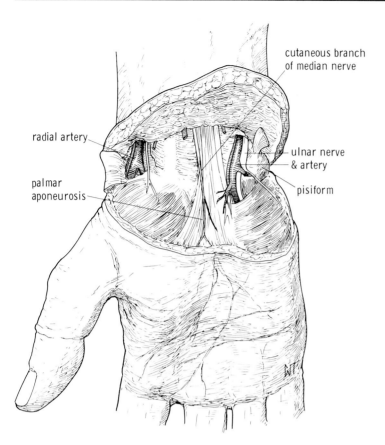

Figure 17-15.   Exposure of the radial and ulnar arteries.

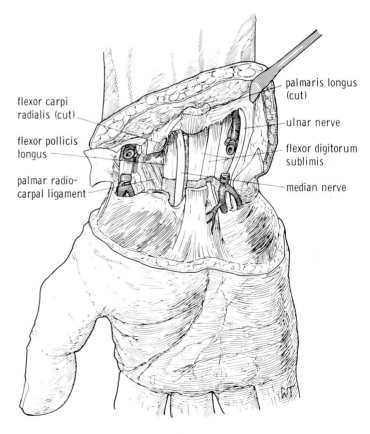

Figure 17-16.   Exposure of the median and ulnar nerves and the carpal canal.

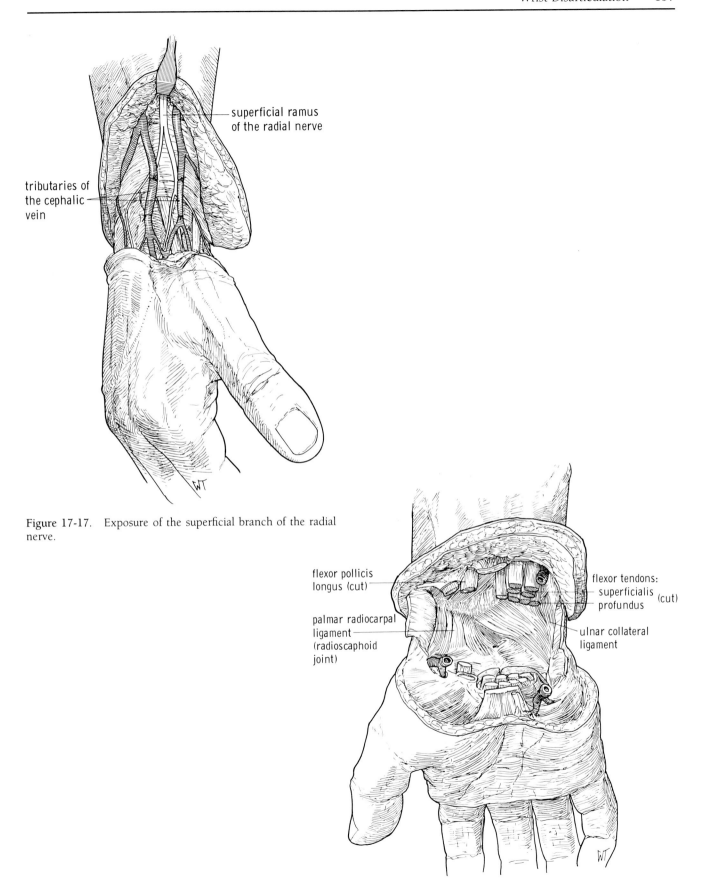

Figure 17-17.   Exposure of the superficial branch of the radial nerve.

superficial ramus of the radial nerve

tributaries of the cephalic vein

flexor pollicis longus (cut)

palmar radiocarpal ligament (radioscaphoid joint)

flexor tendons: superficialis (cut) profundus

ulnar collateral ligament

Figure 17-18.   The wrist is extended and adducted. The palmar radiocarpal ligament provides a landmark for the entry into the radiocarpal joint.

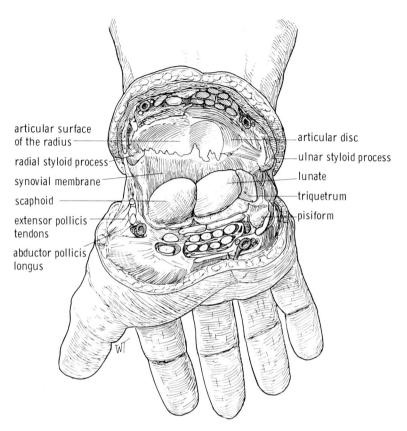

articular surface
of the radius

radial styloid process

synovial membrane

scaphoid

extensor pollicis
tendons

abductor pollicis
longus

articular disc

ulnar styloid process

lunate

triquetrum

pisiform

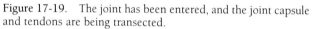

Figure 17-19.   The joint has been entered, and the joint capsule and tendons are being transected.

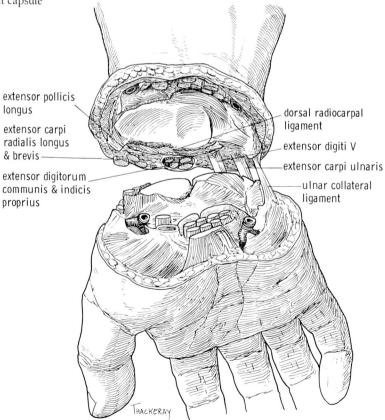

extensor pollicis
longus

extensor carpi
radialis longus
& brevis

extensor digitorum
communis & indicis
proprius

dorsal radiocarpal
ligament

extensor digiti V

extensor carpi ulnaris

ulnar collateral
ligament

Figure 17-20.   Immediately prior to transection of the last remaining structures. The distal radioulnar joint has been preserved.

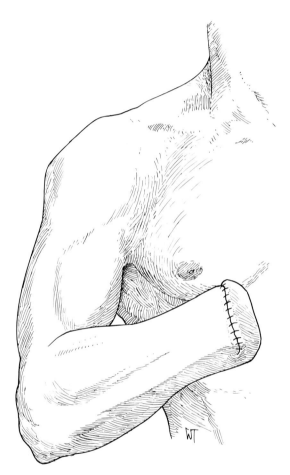

Figure 17-21.   Skin closure is completed.

CHAPTER 18
Amputations Through the Forearm

In the upper extremity, preservation of the elbow is of great importance. In addition a forearm stump of adequate length to allow anchorage of the prosthesis is very desirable. Even if this ideal length cannot be preserved, however, a functioning elbow with a short stump is highly desirable as a power source.

STANDARD BELOW-ELBOW AMPUTATION

Amputation in the lower third of the forearm—desirable as it may be from the standpoint of stump length—is rarely successful. The lack of coverage with well-vascularized soft tissue of adequate thickness is the usual cause for failure. Thus, amputation at this level is attempted mainly in children where the skin flaps are usually sufficient for coverage.

A source of ideal soft tissue coverage starts at the musculotendinous junction of the forearm muscles. Even if a myofascial flap cannot be used to cover the bone end, the musculature surrounding the remnants of the forearm bones will provide enough circulation as long as it is prevented by myodesis from retracting beyond the ends of the bone.

Technique

The patient is placed in the supine position. The involved extremity is prepared and draped, and is abducted on the hand table. The tourniquet is inflated. If equal flaps are chosen, the most proximal points of the skin incision are marked approximately 1 cm distal to the intended level of bone transection on the radial and ulnar side, with the forearm in midposition between pronation and supination. The skin flaps are convex and slightly longer than half the diameter of the forearm at the intended level of bone transection (Fig. 18-1). If myofascial flaps can be obtained, they can be chosen from either both the dorsal and volar side of the forearm (Fig. 18-2), or from one side only—preferably the more muscular volar side. The flaps are tapered in thickness to approximately 2 cm to avoid excessive bulkiness. The bones are transected at the chosen level and beveled (Fig. 18-3). This is particularly important at the subcutaneous border of the ulna, which can create a rather prominent corner and erode the skin. Blood vessels are doubly ligated, and the nerves are dissected free and cut well above the level of amputation. After removal of the tourniquet, further hemostasis is obtained.

A suction drain is placed into the amputation wound, and soft tissue closure is begun by approximating the edges of the myofascial flap with interrupted absorbable sutures (Fig. 18-4). Subcutaneous and skin closure is done with interrupted nonabsorbable sutures (Fig. 18-5).

Where myofascial flaps cannot be fashioned, the musculature should be cut approximately 1.5 to 2 cm below the intended level of bone transection or secured by myodesis. It is more important to maintain the ideal length of the bone stump than to obtain extensive coverage at the stump end. Thus, the skin coverage can be obtained through atypical skin flaps as long as they are well vascularized. Where possible, it is desirable to use the fascia antebrachii for stump coverage.

Figures 18-1 to 18-5.   Standard below-elbow amputation.

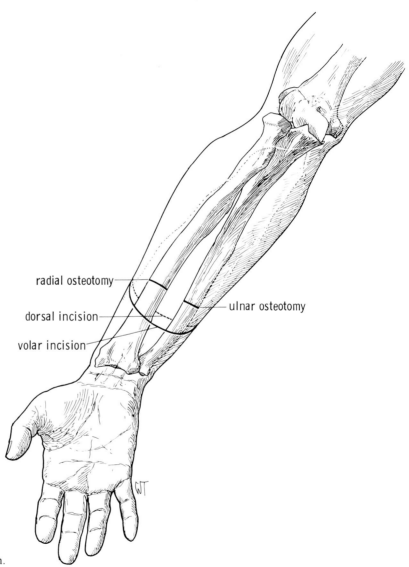

radial osteotomy

ulnar osteotomy

dorsal incision

volar incision

Figure 18-1.   Outline of the skin incision.

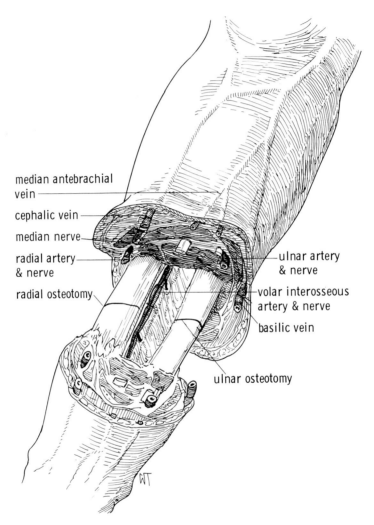

median antebrachial
vein

cephalic vein

median nerve

radial artery
& nerve

radial osteotomy

ulnar artery
& nerve

volar interosseous
artery & nerve

basilic vein

ulnar osteotomy

Figure 18-2. Radius and ulnar are exposed, and the soft tissue
flaps are beveled.

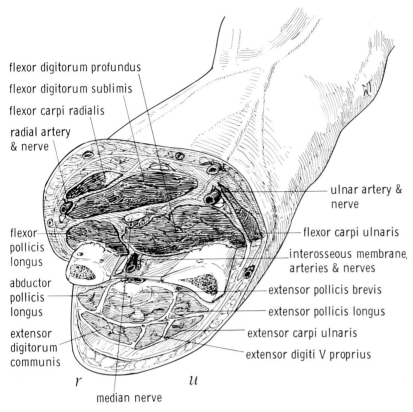

flexor digitorum profundus

flexor digitorum sublimis

flexor carpi radialis

radial artery
& nerve

flexor
pollicis
longus

abductor
pollicis
longus

extensor
digitorum
communis

ulnar artery &
nerve

flexor carpi ulnaris

interosseous membrane,
arteries & nerves

extensor pollicis brevis

extensor pollicis longus

extensor carpi ulnaris

extensor digiti V proprius

median nerve

r   *u*

Figure 18-3.   Amputation through the radius (r) and ulnar (u) has
been completed. Nerves and blood vessels have been ligated.

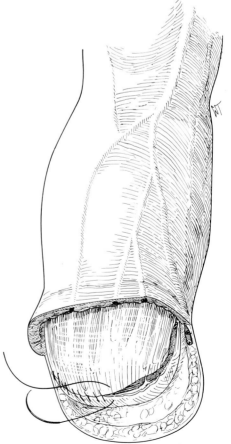

Figure 18-4.   The myofascial flaps are approximated by interrupted sutures.

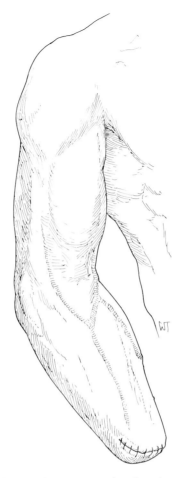

Figure 18-5.   Stump after skin closure.

KRUKENBERG PROCEDURE[1,2]

The aim of the Krukenberg procedure is to provide the patient with grasp, utilizing at the same time the sensation of the skin of the forearm. It changes the forearm itself into a prehensile organ by separating radius and ulna, using them as actively moving tongs. The prerequisites for this procedure, therefore, are presence of adequate length of the forearm bones (15 cm or longer in the adult), good sensation of the skin of the forearm with minimal scarring, and good muscle power. Adequate length of the forearm bones is necessary because of the need for adequate opening at the end of the tongs. No attempt should be made to amputate rudimentary fingers in the case of congenital deformities.

Technique

This procedure is performed under tourniquet control. The involved extremity is prepped and draped free. Another area of the abdomen or thigh is prepped and draped to serve as the donor site for a split thickness graft. The skin incisions are mapped out eccentrically between the forearm bones. On the volar aspect, the incision is placed slightly more toward the radius, whereas on the dorsal surface, the incision is more toward the ulna (Fig. 18-6). Either a single dorsal or a dorsal and a volar V-shaped flap are outlined to provide coverage in the web space between the two branches. The level of this web space is in the area where the pronator teres muscle crosses the interosseous membrane. The fascia antebrachii is opened, and the musculature is divided between the two intended branches (Figs. 18-7 and 18-8). The radial half of the flexor digitorum sublimis and extensor digitorum communis, the flexor carpi radialis, extensor carpi radialis longus and brevis, the brachioradialis, the palmaris longus, the pronator teres, and the extrinsic muscles to the thumb remain with the radius, as do the radial and median nerves. The ulnar half of the flexor digitorum sublimis and extensor digitorum communis, as well as flexor carpi ulnaris and extensor carpi ulnaris with the ulnar nerve, go with the ulna. The pronator quadratus and the flexor digitorum profundus must be excised. If there is too much muscle bulk, the abductor and flexor pollicis longus and extensor pollicis brevis may also be resected, unless these muscles provide power to a single remaining digit.[2]

The tendons of the individual muscles are either sutured into the periosteum or secured with sutures to drill holes in the distal end of the forearm bones (Fig. 18-9). In the growing individual, care is to be taken not to interfere with the distal ulnar or radial physis[4]. With the tongs fully closed, the distal ends of the two branches should touch. Where there is inadequate closure, an osteotomy can be performed to provide apposition.

The interosseous membrane is teased off its ulnar attachment by putting radius and ulna under slight distraction (Fig. 18-8). In this fashion, the interosseous nerve is preserved. Care has to be taken not to interfere with the nerve and blood supply to the pronator teres or with the muscle itself, since it provides the strongest closing mechanism for the tongs and probably prevents subluxation of the radiohumeral joint. Its distal border in the interosseous space provides the landmark for the web space of the tongs.

The tourniquet is now released, and the two branches are covered with skin in such a fashion that scars do not lie in the opposing surfaces. Debulking of the skin flaps and excision of redundant muscle tissue may be necessary to allow primary closure over the branches. The V-shaped flaps are brought into the web space. Frequently, there remains on the flexor surface an open area that requires coverage with a split thickness skin graft (Fig. 18-10).

The spread between the tips of the tongs should be between 6 and 12 cm[5]. By placing fluffed gauze between the branches of the tongs, this opening should be maintained in the dressing. The dressing itself is bulky.

Figures 18-6 to 18-10.   The Krukenberg procedure.

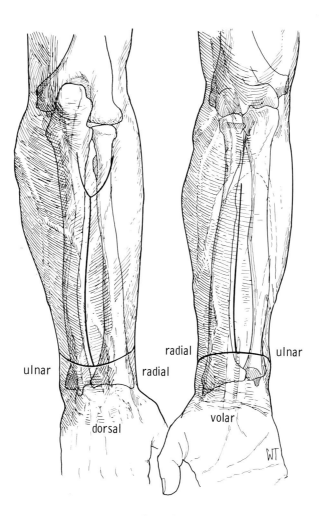

Figure 18-6.   Outline of the skin incisions.

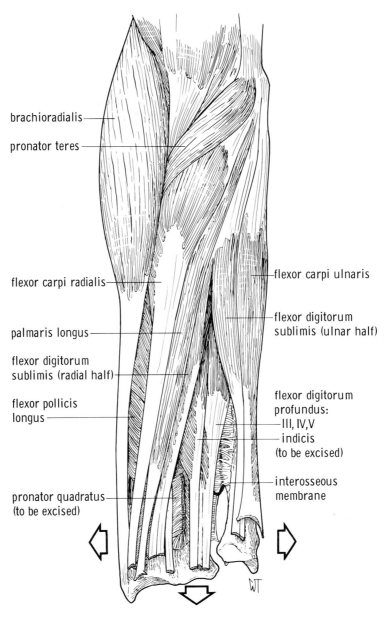

brachioradialis

pronator teres

flexor carpi radialis

palmaris longus

flexor digitorum
sublimis (radial half)

flexor pollicis
longus

pronator quadratus
(to be excised)

flexor carpi ulnaris

flexor digitorum
sublimis (ulnar half)

flexor digitorum
profundus:
III, IV, V
indicis
(to be excised)

interosseous
membrane

Figure 18-7.   Division of the volar musculature between the two branches of the pincers. Pronator quadratus, flexor indicis proprius, and the ulnar portion of the flexor digitorum profundus will be excised.

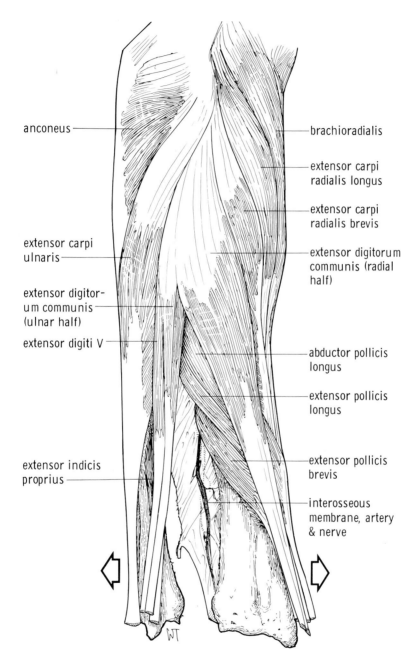

anconeus

brachioradialis

extensor carpi
radialis longus

extensor carpi
radialis brevis

extensor carpi
ulnaris

extensor digitorum
communis (radial
half)

extensor digitor-
um communis
(ulnar half)

extensor digiti V

abductor pollicis
longus

extensor pollicis
longus

extensor indicis
proprius

extensor pollicis
brevis

interosseous
membrane, artery
& nerve

Figure 18-8.   Division of the dorsal forearm musculature between the two
branches. The interosseous membrane is being detached from the ulnar by gently
separating ulnar and radius.

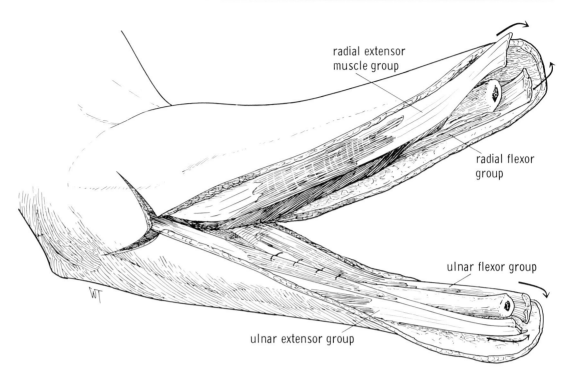

Figure 18-9.   Musculature is attached to the periosteum of the respective forearm bone.

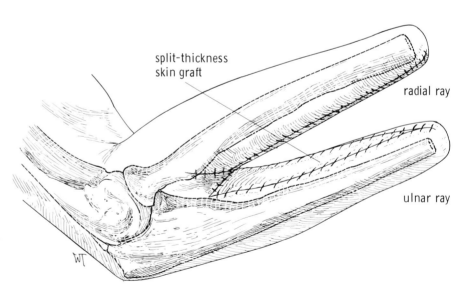

Figure 18-10.   A completed Krukenberg plasty.

Modification

In an attempt to close the skin without grafting and to ensure a distal grasping surface free of scars, S-shaped volar and dorsal incisions have been recom-

mended. Primary closure without skin grafting, however, requires resection of considerable muscle bulk. The recommendation has been to remove palmaris longus, flexor carpi radialis, flexor digitorum sublimis, extensor carpi radialis longus, and brevis and extrinsic thumb muscles.[3]

AMPUTATIONS THROUGH THE FOREARM ABOVE THE IDEAL LEVEL

Some amount of pronation and supination of the arm can be expected with amputations at levels up to the midforearm. Beyond that, the soft tissue mantle of the stump obscures movements of forearm bones. Stumps less than 5 cm present greater problems in prosthetic fitting. It is possible to gain better seating of the prosthesis by resection of the biceps tendon (Fig. 18-11). This can either be done through the amputation wound by undermining the soft tissue covering the stump of the radius, or through a separate transverse incision 2 to 3 cm above the elbow crease. After transection of the tendon of the biceps, approximately 3 cm of the overall length of the tendon is resected (Fig. 18-12).

Figures 18-11 and 18-12.   High below-elbow amputation.

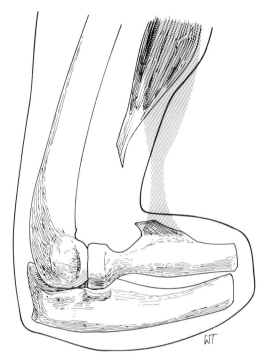

Figure 18-11.   Schematic representation of the biceps tendon transection to gain stump length.

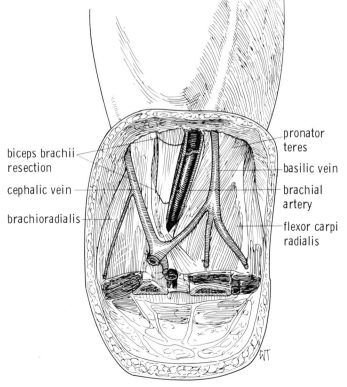

Figure 18-12.   Exposure of the biceps tendon through the amputation wound. The distance of tendon to be resected is indicated.

ELBOW DISARTICULATION

Disarticulation of the forearm through the elbow joint in children is preferable to above-elbow amputation. Preservation of the epiphysis allows commensurate growth between the bone and the soft tissues. Spindling and overgrowth of the diaphysis can be avoided.

Technique

The patient is placed in the supine position and the arm is placed on the arm board. It is prepared and draped. The tournique is inflated. For the posterior incision, the elbow is flexed 90°. A posterior, distally convex skin flap is created from the medial to the lateral epicondyle, with its distal extremity approximately 3 cm distal to the tip of the olecranon (Fig. 18-13). The anterior incision is distally convex, with its most distal part being 2 cm distal to the elbow crease (Fig. 18-13). Atypical flaps can be used; however, it is desirable to maintain as much of the dorsal skin as possible.

After raising the skin flap up to the level of the epicondyles, the anterior part of the elbow is exposed (Fig. 18-14). The lacertus fibrosis is incised from the medial to the lateral side, exposing the flexor muscles. These are transected a the level of the proposed disarticulation, exposing the radial artery and vein and the median nerve (Fig. 18-15). The median nerve is transected well above the level of amputation. Next, after they have been doubly ligated, the veins and artery are transected. On the lateral side of the neurovascular bundle lies the tendon of the biceps brachii; lateral to this is the lateral antebrachial cutaneous nerve. The tendon of the biceps is detached from the radial tubercle; the nerve is treated in the usual fashion. Underneath the biceps tendon, the brachialis muscle is resected from its insertion at the coronoid process (Fig. 18-16). Now the brachialis muscle can be lifted up with the radial nerve coming into view. The nerve is dissected free and transected above the level of the amputation. The brachioradialis muscle, as well as the extensor muscles to the wrist and fingers, are transected 4 to 6 cm below the level of disarticulation, and are beveled in such a fashion that they provide a flap for distal coverage. The anconeus muscle is removed from the lateral epicondyle, and the triceps tendon is separated from the olecranon (Fig. 18-17). In the ulnar groove, the ulnar nerve is now clearly visible. It too is transected well above the level of amputation. At this point, the anterior capsule, medial collateral ligament, and the much weaker lateral collateral ligament can be incised. The elbow can now be slightly overextended, and disarticulation can be completed by incising the rest of the capsule (Fig. 18-18).

The biceps tendon and brachialis tendon are sutured over the trochlea to the triceps tendon (Fig. 18-19). The suction drain is introduced into the wound, and the flap that is fashioned from the extensor muscles is brought medially and sutured to the stump of the flexor muscles (Fig. 18-20). Skin closure is obtained by interrupted sutures (Fig. 18-21).

Figures 18-13 to 18-21.   Elbow disarticulation.

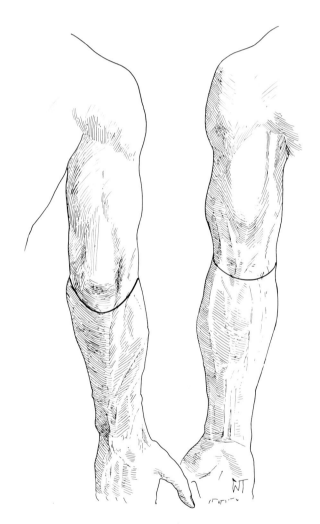

Figure 18-13.   Skin incision.

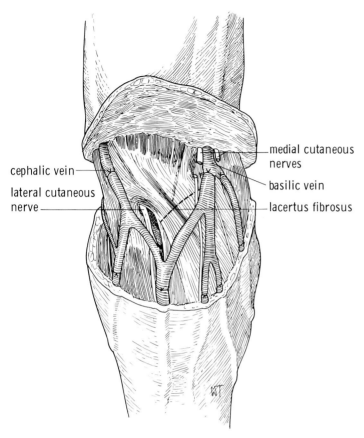

cephalic vein

lateral cutaneous
nerve

medial cutaneous
nerves

basilic vein

lacertus fibrosus

Figure 18-14. Exposure of the subcutaneous structures on the flexor aspect.

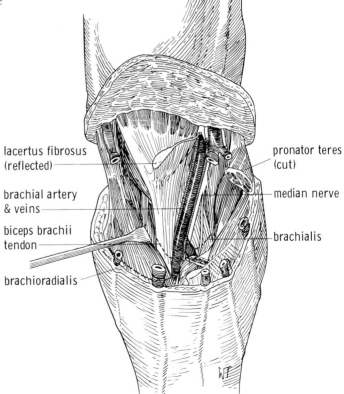

lacertus fibrosus
(reflected)

brachial artery
& veins

biceps brachii
tendon

brachioradialis

pronator teres
(cut)

median nerve

brachialis

Figure 18-15. The lacertus fibrosus has been transected and reflected. The levels of transection of the flexor muscles are indicated.

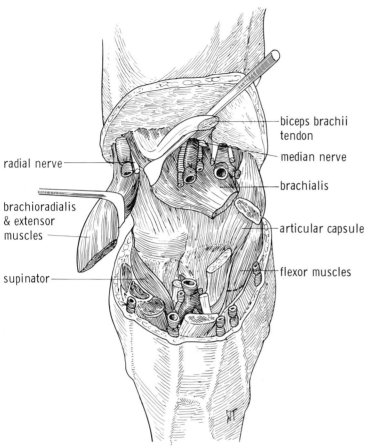

radial nerve

brachioradialis & extensor muscles

supinator

biceps brachii tendon

median nerve

brachialis

articular capsule

flexor muscles

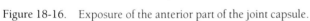

Figure 18-16.   Exposure of the anterior part of the joint capsule.

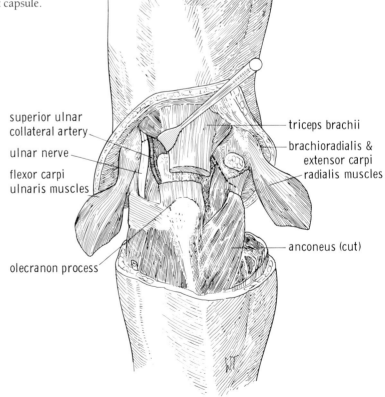

superior ulnar collateral artery

ulnar nerve

flexor carpi ulnaris muscles

olecranon process

triceps brachii

brachioradialis & extensor carpi radialis muscles

anconeus (cut)

Figure 18-17.   Exposure and transection of the posterior structures of the elbow.

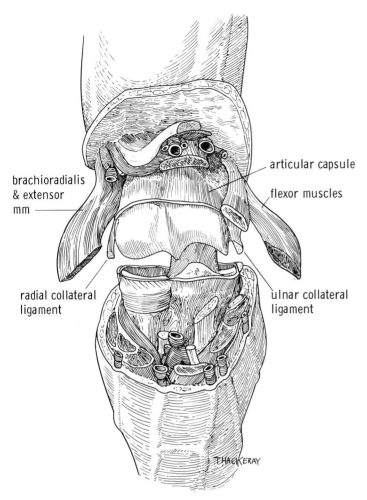

brachioradialis
& extensor
mm

articular capsule

flexor muscles

radial collateral
ligament

ulnar collateral
ligament

Figure 18-18.   Anterior view of the elbow joint after transection
of all soft tissue structures including the joint capsule.

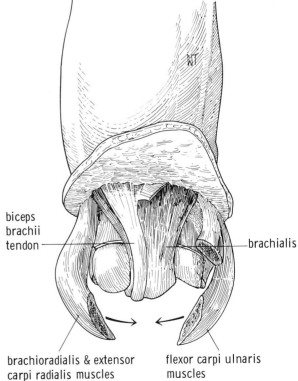

biceps
brachii
tendon

brachialis

brachioradialis & extensor
carpi radialis muscles

flexor carpi ulnaris
muscles

Figure 18-19.   Biceps brachii and brachialis tendons are sutured
to the triceps tendon.

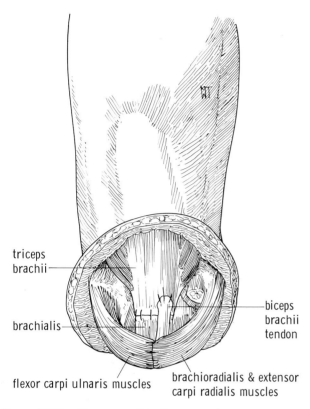

triceps
brachii

brachialis

biceps
brachii
tendon

flexor carpi ulnaris muscles

brachioradialis & extensor
carpi radialis muscles

Figure 18-20. The stump of the flexor muscles is approximated to the stump of the brachial radiali and the extensor muscles.

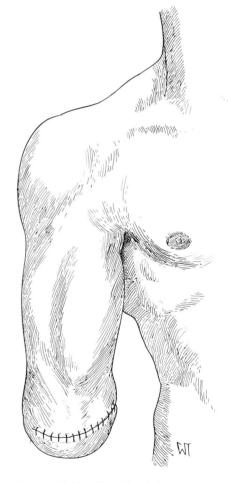

Figure 18-21. Completed skin closure.

References

1. Ritsila V, Kivilaakso R: Modification of Krukenberg kineplastic operation. *Ann Chirurgiae Gynaecologiae* 65:338–341, 1976.

2. Swanson AB, Swanson G deG: The Krukenberg procedure in the juvenile amputee. *Clin Orthopaedics* 148:55–61, 1980.

3. Nathan PA, Trung NB: The Krukenberg operation: A modified technique avoiding skin grafts. *J Hand Surg* 2:127–130, 1977.

4. Harrison SH, Mayou B: Bilateral Krukenberg operations in a young child. *Br J Plastic Surg* 30:171–173, 1977.

5. Tubiana R, Krukenberg's Operation. *Orthopedic Clin North Am* 12(4):819–826, 1981.

CHAPTER 19
Above the Elbow Amputation

This area of amputation extends from the transcondylar level to the gleno-humeral joint. It allows adequate soft tissue coverage for the stump end. If the stump of the humerus is short enough, easy fitting with a standard prosthetic elbow joint is possible. However, the thick layer of soft tissue surrounding the humerus allows considerable movement of the socket of the prosthesis. In addition, the shoulder rotation becomes less effective because of the malleability of the soft tissue mantle. Therefore, special procedures have been devised to improve the rotation.[4]

TRANSCONDYLAR AMPUTATION

In an attempt to use the greater width at the distal end of the humerus to transmit internal and external rotation at the shoulder to the socket of the prosthesis, transcondylar amputation can be attempted. The advantage of the amputation is weighted against the fact that the stump is of considerable length, and that special efforts must be made to accommodate the elbow mechanism of the prosthesis.

Technique

The patient is placed in the supine position, and the arm is placed on the arm board. The skin incision is placed in such a way that from a line connecting the midpoints of the medial and lateral epicondyle, the anterior and posterior skin flaps of equal length are formed (Fig. 19-1). Medially, in the anterior part of the wound, the lacertus fibrosis is detached. Under it, the median nerve, brachial artery, and brachial vein are found (Figs. 19-2 and 19-3). The vein and artery are doubly ligated and transected; the median nerve is dissected free to about 2 cm above the intended amputation site and transected. Further to the medial side, the wrist and finger flexors are detached from the medial epicondyle. On the lateral side, the biceps and brachialis tendons are detached from their respective insertions. Upon lifting the brachioradialis muscle, the radial nerve comes into view and can be dissected free to be severed further proximally. The brachioradialis muscle and part of the extensor muscles of the wrist and fingers are severed 5 to 6 cm distally to the lateral epicondyle. They are beveled to be used as coverage for the distal surface of the stump of the bone (Fig. 19-4). The triceps tendon is then detached from the olecranon, and the ulnar nerve is dissected free to be severed proximally from the amputation site. The anterior part of the capsule is incised. Then, with the elbow in 20° flexion, the humeral condyle is transected through its widest part (Fig. 19-4). This usually leaves a small remnant of the capitulum humeri and of the posterior part of the trochlea humeri. These have to be smoothed off together, with the sharp edges of the bone at the level of the section.

The triceps tendon is then sutured to the brachialis and biceps tendon (Figure 19-5). A suction drain is inserted into the wound, and the thin flap of the extensor muscles is sutured over the sectioned end of the bone to the medial epicondyle. Subcutaneous tissue and skin are closed.

Figures 19-1 to 19-5.   Transcondylar amputation.

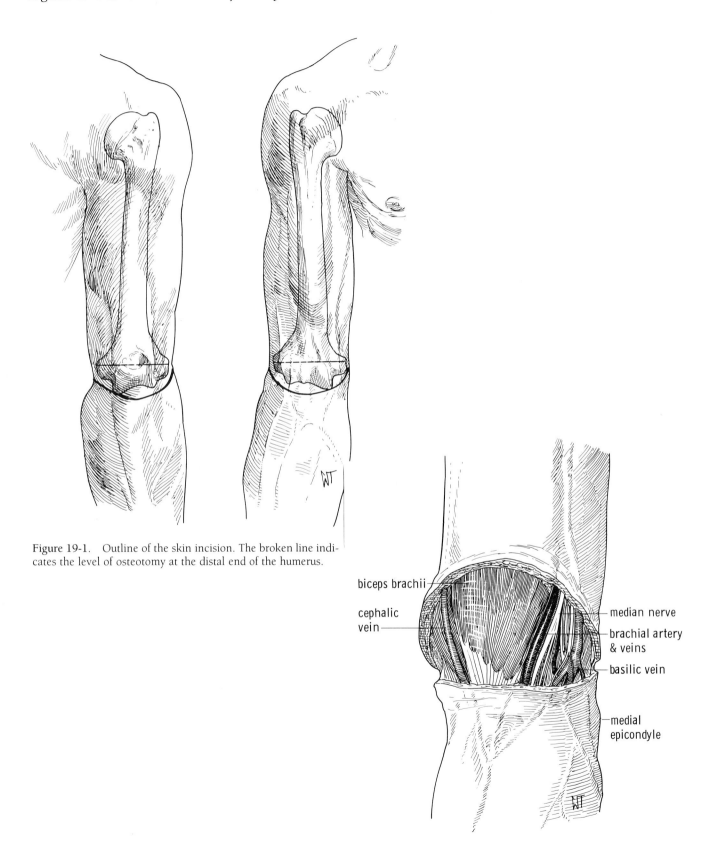

Figure 19-1.   Outline of the skin incision. The broken line indicates the level of osteotomy at the distal end of the humerus.

biceps brachii

cephalic vein

median nerve

brachial artery & veins

basilic vein

medial epicondyle

Figure 19-2.   The median nerve and brachial vessels are found at the medial border of the biceps.

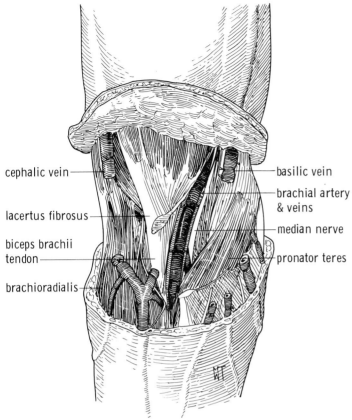

cephalic vein

lacertus fibrosus

biceps brachii
tendon

brachioradialis

basilic vein

brachial artery
& veins

median nerve

pronator teres

Figure 19-3. The artery and nerve have been ligated and transected.

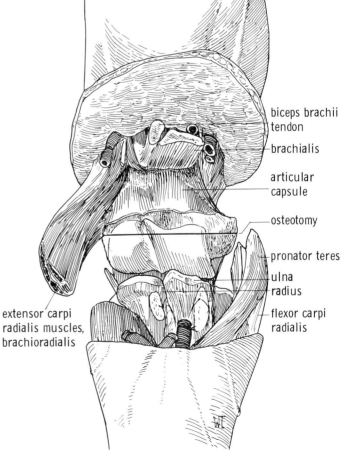

biceps brachii
tendon

brachialis

articular
capsule

osteotomy

pronator teres

ulna
radius

flexor carpi
radialis

extensor carpi
radialis muscles,
brachioradialis

Figure 19-4. The elbow joint has been entered after transection of the surrounding soft tissue. The solid line indicates the level of the transcondylar osteotomy.

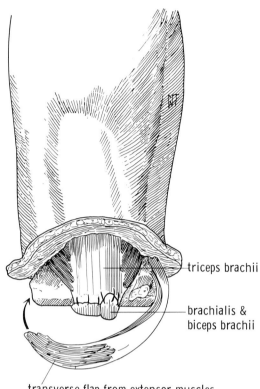

triceps brachii

brachialis &
biceps brachii

transverse flap from extensor muscles

Figure 19-5.   Brachialis and biceps brachii tendons have been sutured to the triceps tendon. The stump of the muscles arising from the lateral epicondyle is being placed over the surface of the osteotomy site.

SUPRACONDYLAR AMPUTATION

Beyond the humeral condyles, the tubular shape of the humeral diaphysis allows considerable movement between the bone and the surrounding soft tissue. Therefore, the rotatory movements in the shoulder are transmitted only partially and weakened in their strength. However, the supracondylar amputation provides a long and well-muscled stump, which allows good anchorage of the prosthetic socket.[5]

Technique

The patient is placed in the supine position with a sandbag under the shoulder on the affected side. The skin incision is of either equal anterior and posterior flaps or atypical flaps as long as circulation is maintained. If equal anterior and posterior flaps are selected, the incision starts at the midlateral line at the level of the intended transection of the bone; it curves distally and anteriorly in a semicircular line over a distance slightly more than the radius of the upper arm at the level of the intended amputation. The incision is continued to the midmedial line at the level of the transection of the bone. An equally shaped skin flap is created on the posterior aspect (Fig. 19-6). The flexor muscles are divided at a slight angle to the bone, with the anterior aspect being somewhat longer than the central parts (Figs. 19-7 and 19-8). Most of the major nerves and vessels now come into view. The median nerve, and brachial artery and veins are found medial to the biceps tendon. The artery and veins are ligated and severed, and the median nerve is transected at a higher level. Slightly posteriorly to those structures are the medial antebrachial cutaneous nerve and the vena basilica. Further laterally, between the biceps and brachialis muscles, lies the lateral cutaneous antebrachial nerve. Between the brachioradialis and the brachialis muscles, the trunk of the radial nerve and the arteria profunda brachii are found. On the lateral side of the brachioradialis, the dorsal antebrachial cutaneous nerve is found. Now, the triceps is detached above the olecranon. Lifting the triceps from the bone brings into view the ulnar nerve on its medial edge. This nerve is also dissected free and transected. The flexor muscles are elevated from the humerus and pushed back approximately 2 cm. The supracondylar level of the humerus is found, and the bone is severed (Fig. 19-9). After release of the tour-

niquet, hemostasis has to be secured because of the various collateral branches around the elbow.

Closure begins with insertion of a suction drain into the amputation wound. The triceps flap is brought forward and sutured into the anterior part of the fascia brachii. The skin flaps are then approximated (Fig. 19-10).

Figures 19-6 to 19-10.   Supracondylar amputation.

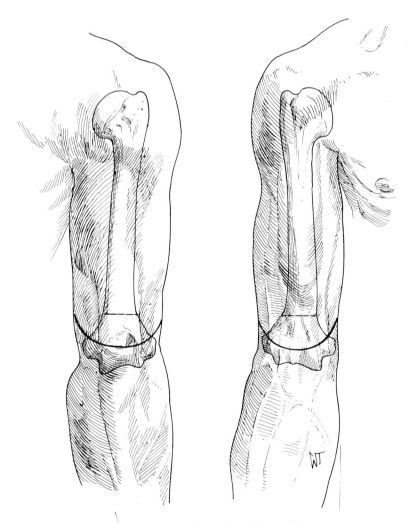

Figure 19-6.   Outline of the skin incision.

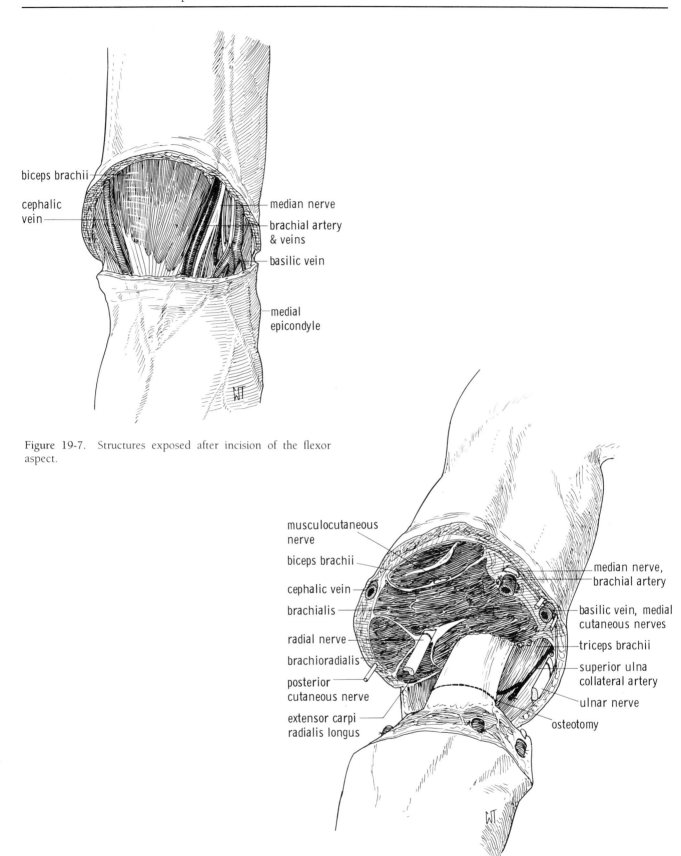

Figure 19-7. Structures exposed after incision of the flexor aspect.

Figure 19-8. The soft tissues on the flexor aspect have been transected, and muscles have been beveled. The broken line indicates the level of the osteotomy.

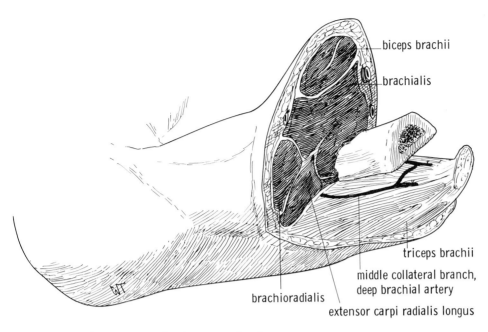

biceps brachii

brachialis

triceps brachii

middle collateral branch,
deep brachial artery

brachioradialis

extensor carpi radialis longus

Figure 19-9.   The amputation has been completed.

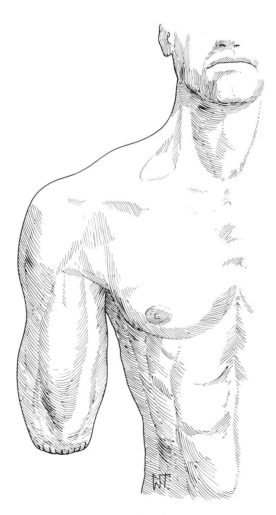

Figure 19-10.   Skin closure.

ABOVE THE ELBOW AMPUTATIONS PROXIMAL TO THE SUPRACONDYLAR LEVEL

If an amputation proximal to the supracondylar area must be performed, the surgeon must consider that sufficient length of the bony stump is necessary to anchor a prosthesis. A minimum of 5 cm below the anterior axillary fold is usually necessary for adequate anchorage of the socket. Ideal soft tissue coverage may have to be sacrificed to maintain length of the humeral stump. Retraction of the musculature leads to a protruding bony stump that is only covered by skin and subcutaneous tissue. Thus, approximation of the fascia and, possibly, myofascial flaps is important[2,3].

Technique

The patient is placed in the supine position with a sandbag under the shoulder on the affected side. The tourniquet is inflated. The intended level of transection of the humerus is marked on the skin in the midmedial and midlateral lines. From these points, anterior and posterior skin flaps are outlined. These flaps are slightly longer than the radius of the humerus at the level of amputation (Fig. 19-11). On the medial aspect of the upper arm, the neurovascular structures are identified and dissected free above the level of the bony transection. The brachial artery and veins, as well as the basilic vein, are doubly ligated and transected. The median, ulnar, and medial antebrachial cutaneous nerves are transected proximal to the site of soft tissue closure (Figs. 19-12 and 19-13). The muscles of the anterior and posterior compartment are cut so that they are beveled to allow soft tissue coverage of the stump end, yet loose skin closure (Fig. 19-14). The radial nerve is treated in the usual manner. The bone is then transected (Fig. 19-15).

The tourniquet is deflated, and hemostasis is obtained. The subcutaneous tissue is closed with interrupted absorbable sutures over the drain (Fig. 19-16). Skin closure is done with interrupted nonabsorbable sutures (Fig. 19-17).

Improvement of Rotation[1]

In an attempt to use the shoulder rotation, a flexion ostetomy has been recommended at the distal end of the stump of the humerus (Fig. 19-18). It is suitable in long or medium-length above-elbow stumps above the level of the condyles. It can be done as a primary procedure at the time of the amputation, or as a secondary procedure. In the latter case, it is suitable in those stumps with bony overgrowth. Depending on the length of the stump, an opening or closing wedge osteotomy can be performed. The procedure is suitable for children as well as adults. In the child, minimal fixation with a Kirschner wire is followed by rapid healing of the bone. In the adult, a more formal fixation with a cortical compression screw is required.

If angulation osteotomy is done at the time of amputation, the skin incision is extended in the midlateral line to a level of approximately 7 to 10 cm above the distal end of the stump of the humerus. In the child, the periosteum is opened only anteriorly or posteriorly, depending on whether a closing or opening wedge is intended. In the case of a closing wedge osteotomy, the anterior half of the cortex of the humerus is transected 4 or 5 cm above the distal end of the humeral stump. In the older child, a small wedge has to be removed. A greenstick fracture is produced in the rest of the cortical bone. A desired angle of 70 to 80° is produced and fixed in this position with a Kirschner wire. In the case of an opening wedge osteotomy, the posterior half of the cortex is transected, and the greenstick fracture is produced through the anterior part of the cortical bone.

In the adult, a more formal wedge removal of 70 to 80° has to be carried out, and the two fragments have to be held in place by a cortical screw. Fragments can be held in place temporarily with a Kirschner wire. Further maintenance of the position can be obtained by application of the postoperative rigid dressing.

If the osteotomy is done as a secondary procedure, the approach is through an anterolateral or dorsolateral incision over the intended osteotomy site, depending upon whether a closing or an opening wedge osteotomy is planned.

Figures 19-11 to 19-18.   Diaphyseal amputation of the humerus.

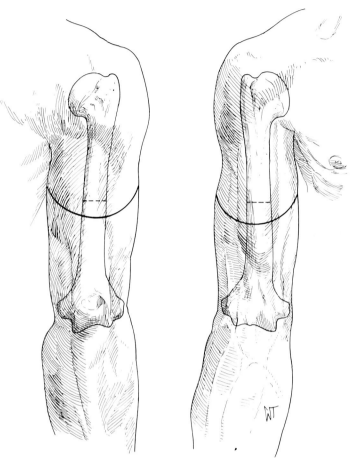

Figure 19-11.   Outline of the skin incision. The broken line indicates the level of bony transection.

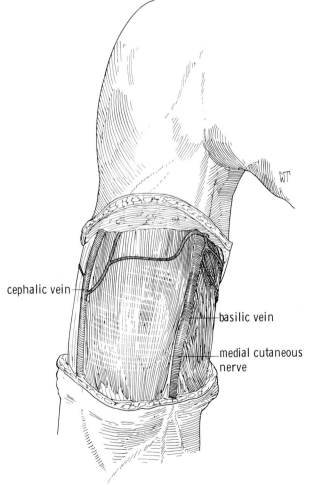

cephalic vein

basilic vein

medial cutaneous
nerve

Figure 19-12.   The superficial veins on the flexor aspect of the upper arm are exposed.

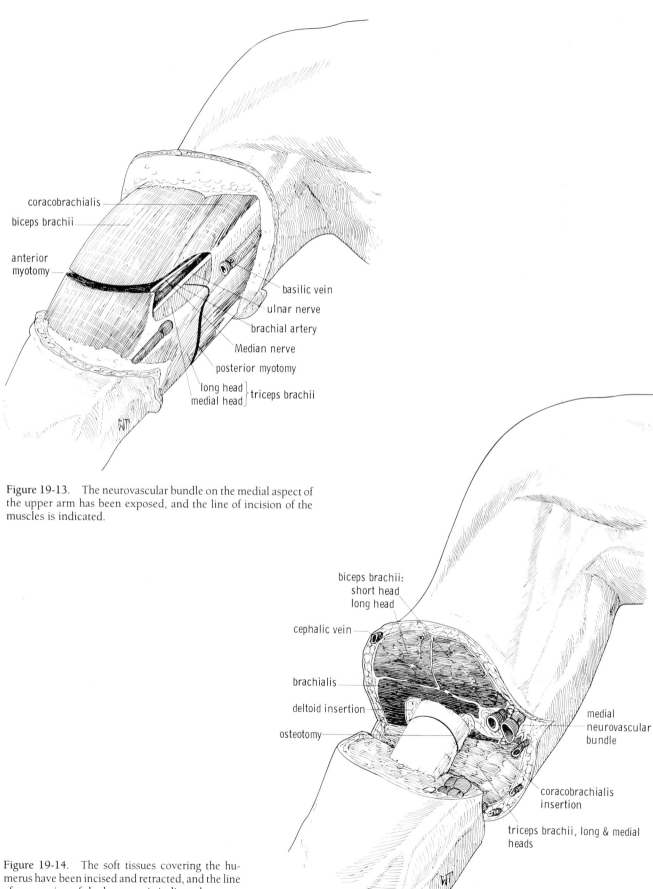

Figure 19-13.   The neurovascular bundle on the medial aspect of the upper arm has been exposed, and the line of incision of the muscles is indicated.

Figure 19-14.   The soft tissues covering the humerus have been incised and retracted, and the line of transection of the humerus is indicated.

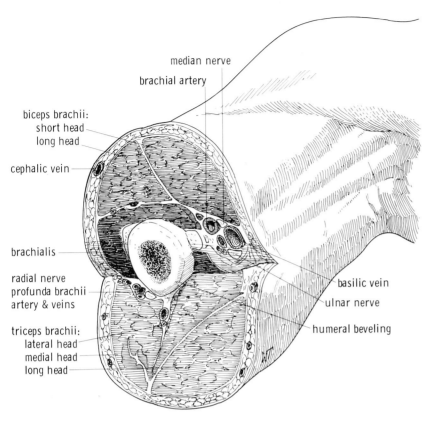

median nerve

brachial artery

biceps brachii:
    short head
    long head

cephalic vein

brachialis

radial nerve
profunda brachii
artery & veins

triceps brachii:
    lateral head
    medial head
    long head

basilic vein

ulnar nerve

humeral beveling

Figure 19-15. The amputation is completed, and beveled soft tissue flaps are ready for closure.

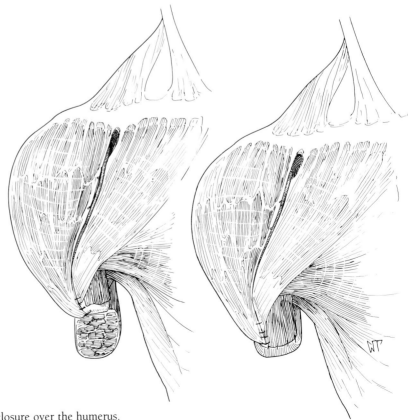

Figure 19-16. Schematic outline of the muscle closure over the humerus.

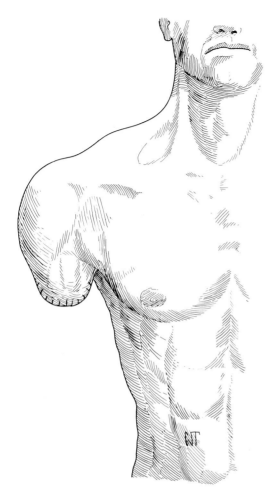

Figure 19-17.   Skin closure has been completed.

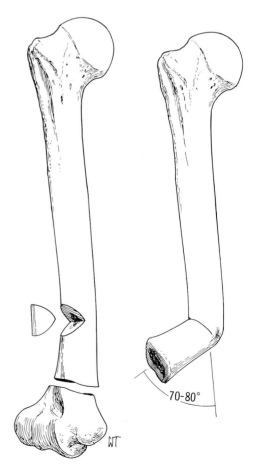

Figure 19-18.   Flexion osteotomy of the distal end of the humerus to improve rotation of the humerus.

AMPUTATION THROUGH THE PROXIMAL END OF THE DIAPHYSIS AND THE PROXIMAL METAPHYSIS OF THE HUMERUS

Even above the minimal level for anchorage of the prosthesis, maintenance of a short humeral stump and shoulder joint are important for the patient. The contour of the shoulder can be maintained, which makes selection of suits and dresses easier. Therefore, if there is a choice between disarticulation of the shoulder through the glenoid fossa and amputation through the upper end of the diaphysis of the humerus, the latter is preferable — even though the remnant of the humerus will not serve as an anchorage for a functional above-elbow prosthesis. For prosthetic fitting, this amputation has to be treated as a shoulder disarticulation.

Technique

The skin incision follows the outline of the deltoid muscle with a margin of approximately 1.5 cm, starting at the tip of the coracoid process of the scapula and ending at the posterior axillary fold. The medial part of the skin incision runs from the anterior to the posterior axillary fold through the axilla (Fig. 19-19).

The neurovascular bundle is exposed after the pectoralis major has been transected close to its insertion into the humerus (Figs. 19-20 and 19-21). Artery and vein are doubly ligated, where they pass under the coracoid process. In severing the nerves, care is to be taken to transect the posterior fascicle distally to the axillary nerve, since it supplies the innervation to the deltoid muscle and the area of the skin overlying it. The deltoid muscle is severed close to its insertion into the humerus and lifted up together with the overlying skin. Under it, the two heads of the biceps and the coracobrachialis muscle come into view. These are transected 2 or 3 cm below the intended level of bone transection. Posteriorly, the latissimus dorsi and teres major muscles are transected near their insertion into the humerus. The long head of the triceps is cut 2 or 3 cm below the intended level of bone transection and beveled (Fig. 19-22). The bone is transected at or near the level of the surgical neck (Fig. 19-23).

Closure is started after remnants of the triceps, biceps, coracobrachialis, and deltoid have been beveled sufficiently. The proximal end of the biceps and coracobrachialis are sutured over the end of the humerus to the triceps. The tendon of the pectoralis major is inserted into the combined muscle mass of these three muscles (Fig. 19-24). A suction drain is inserted into the amputation wound, and the distal end of the deltoid is sutured as a second layer over the soft tissue layer at the distal end of the humerus. The skin edges are approximated (Fig. 19-25).

Figures 19-19 to 19-25.   Amputation through the proximal end of the diaphysis and the proximal metaphysis of the humerus.

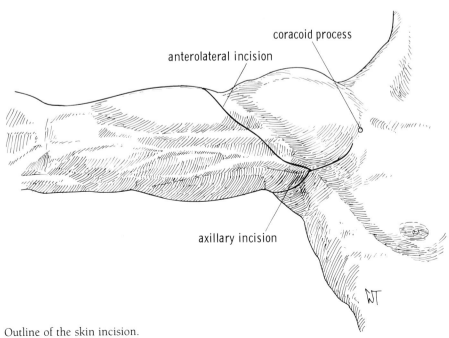

Figure 19-19.   Outline of the skin incision.

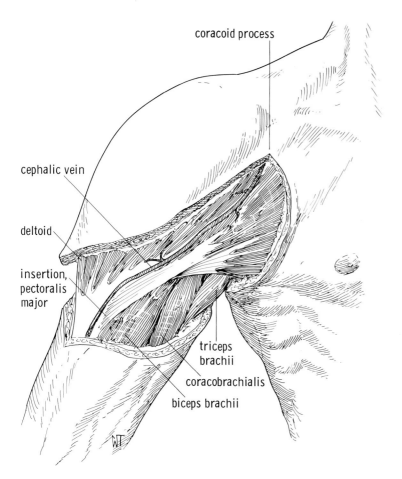

coracoid process

cephalic vein

deltoid

insertion,
pectoralis
major

triceps
brachii

coracobrachialis

biceps brachii

Figure 19-20.   Exposure of the pectoralis major muscle.

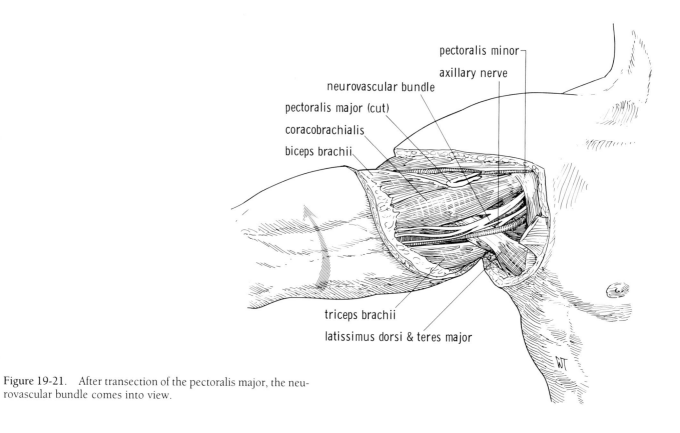

pectoralis minor

axillary nerve

neurovascular bundle

pectoralis major (cut)

coracobrachialis

biceps brachii

triceps brachii

latissimus dorsi & teres major

Figure 19-21.   After transection of the pectoralis major, the neurovascular bundle comes into view.

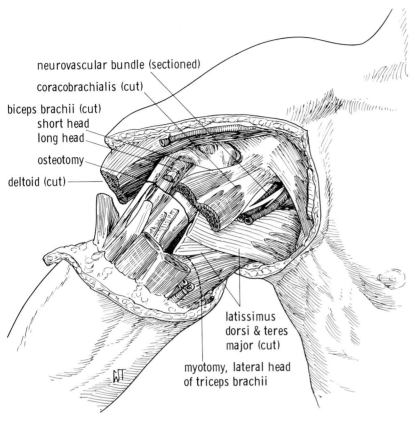

neurovascular bundle (sectioned)

coracobrachialis (cut)

biceps brachii (cut)
short head
long head

osteotomy

deltoid (cut)

latissimus
dorsi & teres
major (cut)

myotomy, lateral head
of triceps brachii

Figure 19-22. The muscles in the anterior part of the exposure have been transected. The neurovascular bundle has been cut and ligated. The solid line indicates the level of amputation through the bone.

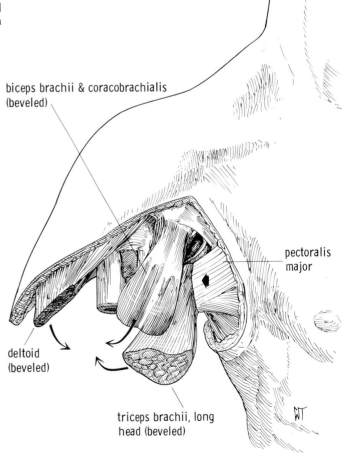

biceps brachii & coracobrachialis
(beveled)

pectoralis
major

deltoid
(beveled)

triceps brachii, long
head (beveled)

Figure 19-23. The amputation has been completed.

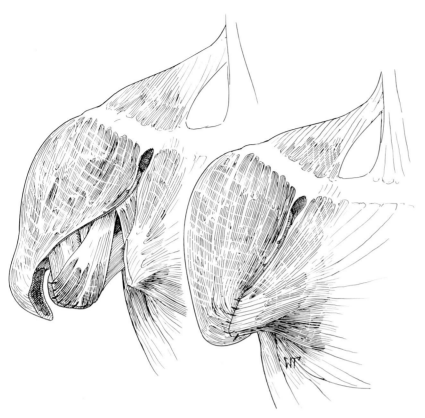

Figure 19-24. Schematic representation of the myoplasty over the end of the bony stump.

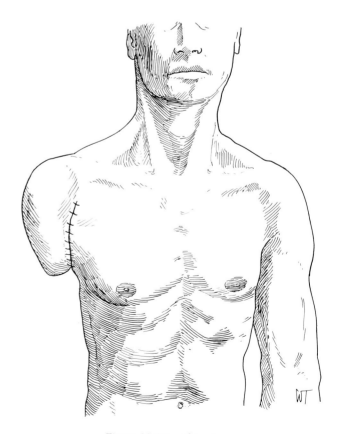

Figure 19-25. Skin closure.

SHOULDER DISARTICULATION

The contour of the shoulder can be preserved to some extend by saving the scapula and clavicle. Coverage of the exposed glenoid fossa can be obtained either by suturing the deltoid muscle over it, or by using the muscles originating from the anterior and posterior surface of the scapula for coverage. This type of coverage, however, will not disguise the sharp projection of the acromium, the acromioclavicular joint, and the concavity right below it (see Fig. 19-32).

Technique

From a supine position, the patient is tilted to the unaffected side at an angle of 40 or 50°. The incision starts at the coracoid process, and parallels the margin of the deltoid muscle with about one finger breadth to spare. It proceeds to the posterior axillary fold. With the arm abducted, the incision is continued through the axilla from the posterior to the anterior axillary fold (Fig. 19-26).

Through the anterior part of the incision, the pectoralis major is identified, sectioned close to the humerus, and retracted medially. Opening the space between the pectoralis minor and the coracobrachialis muscle brings into view the neurovascular bundle (Fig. 19-27). The axillary artery and vein are transected, after clamping on both sides, and then doubly ligated. Upon retraction of the pectoralis minor medially, the thoracoacromial artery can be identified and ligated as well. Gentle retraction of the pectoralis minor and the transected vessels leads to identification of the neural elements, which are transected following ligation. The axillary nerve is spared. The proximal stump of the nerves will be covered by the pectoralis minor.

The coracobrachialis and the short head of the biceps are transected through the tendinous portion close to the coracoid process (Fig. 19-28). The deltoid muscle is lifted off the shaft of the humerus and cut 2 or 3 inches above its insertion. It can now be lifted posterosuperiorly without undue stress on the axillary nerve. By externally rotating the shoulder, the anterior part of the capsule of the shoulder joint can be opened. Further distally, the subscapularis, latissimus dorsi, and teres major tendons are transected. By gradual internal rotation, the superior part of the capsule (with the tendon of the long head of the biceps and the supraspinatus muscle) and the posterior part of the capsule (with the infraspinatus and teres minor muscles) are transected. At the posteroinferior margin of the glenoid fossa, the long head of the triceps can be severed. The transection of the inferior part of the capsule completes the amputation of the upper extremity (Fig. 19-29).

Hemostasis is completed. The tendons of the pectoralis major, teres major, and subscapularis muscles are sutured over the glenoid fossa to the posterior part of the capsule and to the tendons of the supraspinatus, infraspinatus, and teres minor. This provides some amount of bulk to fill in the cavity under the deltoid coverage (Fig. 19-30). The inferior margin of the deltoid is sutured to the inferior part of the capsule (Fig. 19-30). Prior to closing the skin, an attempt should be made to remove all axillary hair by excising sufficient amounts of axillary skin. However, this should only be done if there is enough skin from the lateral aspect of the shoulder available for closure without tension. A suction drain is inserted under the deltoid. The subcutaneous tissue is closed with interrupted absorbable sutures, and the skin is closed with interrupted nonabsorbable sutures (Figs. 19-31 and 19-32).

Figures 19-26 to 19-32.   Shoulder disarticulation (glenohumeral amputation).

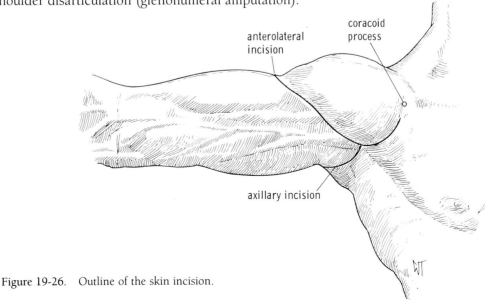

Figure 19-26.   Outline of the skin incision.

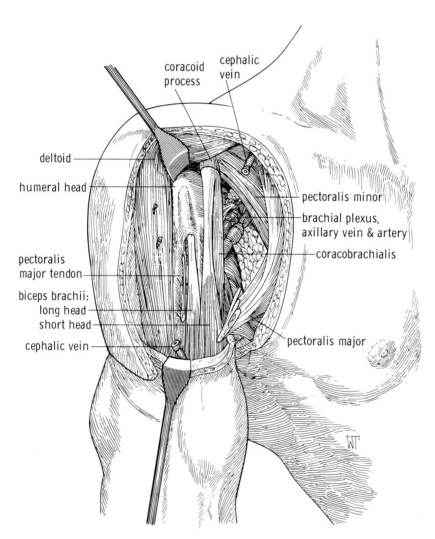

Figure 19-27. The pectoralis major tendon has been transected, the brachial vein and artery ligated.

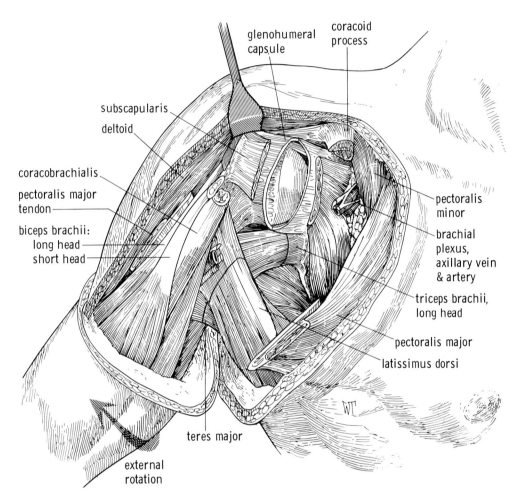

glenohumeral
capsule

coracoid
process

subscapularis

deltoid

coracobrachialis

pectoralis major
tendon

biceps brachii:
long head
short head

pectoralis
minor

brachial
plexus,
axillary vein
& artery

triceps brachii,
long head

pectoralis major

latissimus dorsi

teres major

external
rotation

Figure 19-28.   After transection of the brachial plexus and the tendons of the anterior shoulder muscles, the gleno-humeral capsule can be opened anteriorly.

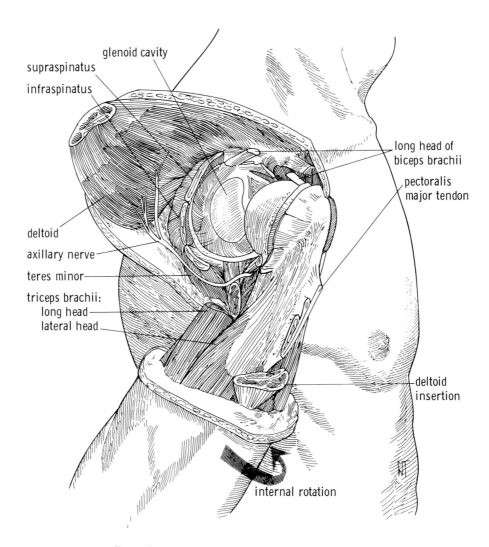

Figure 19-29.   All muscles around the shoulder have been transected. The capsule of the shoulder joint has been opened circumferentially. The axiliary nerve is intact.

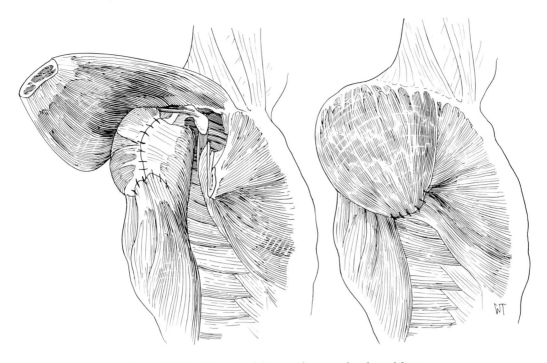

Figure 19-30.   Closure of the muscles over the glenoid fossa.

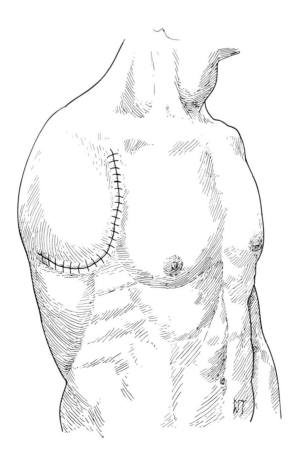

Figure 19-31.   Skin closure as seen from laterally.

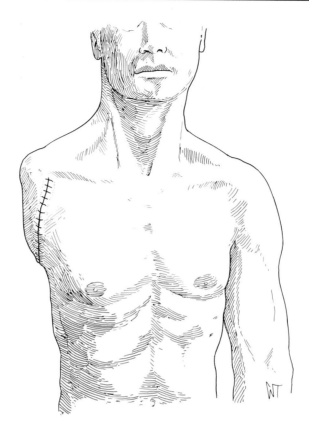

Figure 19-32.   The shoulder disarticulation leaves the involved shoulder narrower and with a sharp projection of the acromioclavicular joint laterally.

References

1. Marquardt E, Neff G: The angulation osteotomy of above-elbow stumps. *Clin Orthopaedics* 104:232–238, 1974.
2. Baumgartner RF: Surgery of arm and forearm amputations. *Orthopaedic Clin North Am* 12(4):805–817, 1981.
3. Elgar F: Amputatio humeri osteoplastica et antebrachii tenoplastica. *Arch klinischer Chirurgie* 88:240–260, 1909.
4. Steinbach TV: Upper limb amputation. *Prog Surg* 16:224–248, 1978
5. Tooms RE: Amputation surgery in the upper extremity. *Orthopaedic Clin North Am* 3(2):383–395, 1972.

CHAPTER 20
Forequarter Amputation

Forequarter amputation consists of the removal of almost half of the shoulder girdle, together with the involved upper extremity. This interscapulothoracic amputation is done almost exclusively for the eradication of malignancies when the tumor involves the entire upper extremity or structures in the immediate vicinity of the shoulder joint. The anterior and posterior approach with the standard skin flaps will be described. However, because of the varying location of the tumors, inventiveness in the shaping of atypical skin flaps may become necessary.[1]

POSTERIOR APPROACH

Technique[2-4]

After induction of general anesthesia, the patient is turned on his or her sound side. The involved upper extremity with the adjacent side of the neck and hemithorax is prepared and draped. The skin incision starts just laterally to the sternoclavicular joint, continues laterally along the clavicle to the acromioclavicular joint, and from there posteriorly along the lateral border to the inferior angle of the scapula (Fig. 20-1). In muscular and overweight people, it may become necessary to curve the incision medially to raise a flap large enough for easy access to the medial border of the scapula. This flap consists of the skin and full thickness of the subcutaneous tissue. It is raised to the medial border of the scapula. The latissimus dorsi muscle is cut (Fig. 20-2). The trapezius muscle is incised close to its spinal border. Under it, the levator scapulae and rhomboid muscles come into view, as well as the transverse cervical artery (Fig. 20-3). The latter is ligated and transected. Thereafter, the muscles are divided close to the me-

dial border of the scapula. By elevating the medial border of the scapula slightly, the transverse scapula artery comes into view (Fig. 20-4). It is ligated and transected. By further elevating the scapula, the serratus anterior muscle can be divided. Depending upon the location of the tumor, this may have to be done further anteriorly.

Moving the scapula anteriorly puts stress upon the subclavian artery and vein, and on the brachial plexus, which appear now in the superior part of the wound. Access to the nerves and vessels can be improved by transecting the omohyoid muscle and by removal of the middle third of the clavicle. The axillary artery and vein are now divided between double ligations, and so is the brachial plexus close to the neck (Fig. 20-5).

The anterior part of the incision is now completed by continuing straight down from the middle of the clavicle through the deltopectoral groove to the anterior axillary line. Curving the incision posteriorly, it meets the posterior limb of the incision somewhat medially to the posterior axillary line (Fig. 20-1). Depending upon the location of the tumor, the pectoralis major and minor muscles are divided closer to the arm or further toward the trunk (Fig. 20-6). Completion of the anterior part of the skin incision, in a slightly medially curved line from the acromioclavicular joint interiorly, and of the posterior incision are the last steps before removal of the extremity.

The remaining stumps of the transected muscles are approximated where possible. Otherwise, they are secured to the soft tissue of the thoracic wall (Fig. 20-7). The skin flaps are fashioned in such a way that there is no redundant tissue (Fig. 20-8). Suction drains are introduced into the wound bed. The subcutaneous tissue is approximated with absorbable sutures. The skin edges are brought together with interrupted nonabsorbable sutures.

Figures 20-1 to 20-8.   Forequarter amputation, posterior approach.

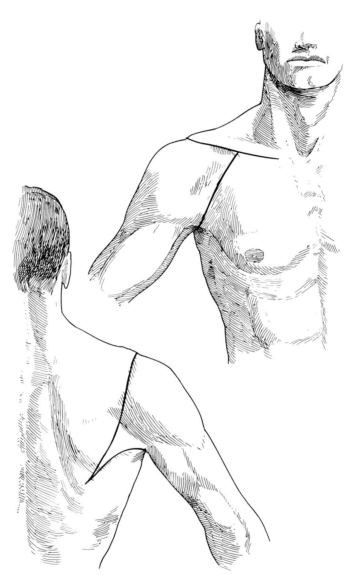

Figure 20-1.   Skin incision.

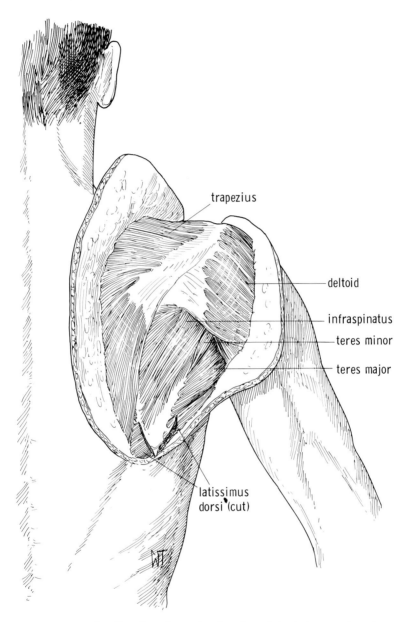

Figure 20-2. Skin flaps have been developed, and the latissimus dorsi has been cut.

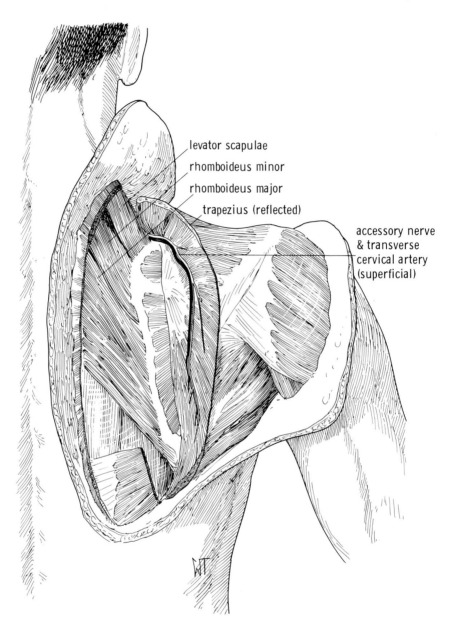

Figure 20-3.   The trapezious muscle has been transected, and the levator scapulae and rhomboideus muscles are in view.

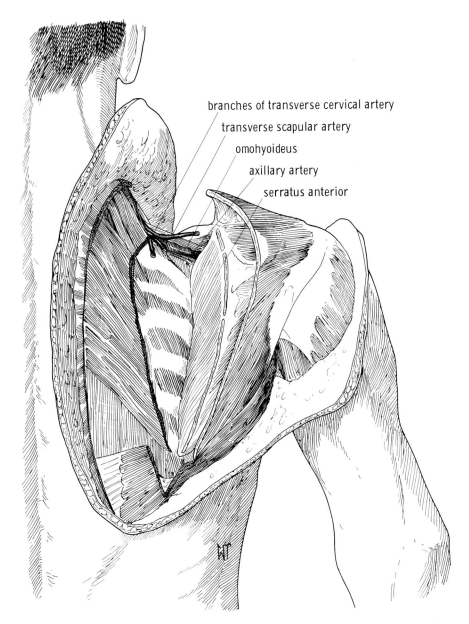

branches of transverse cervical artery
transverse scapular artery
omohyoideus
axillary artery
serratus anterior

Figure 20-4.   The levator scapulae and rhomboideus muscles have been transected. The transverse scapulae artery has been ligated, and the scapula is lifted and pushed forward. The omohyoid muscle and the subclavian artery are in the upper corner of the wound.

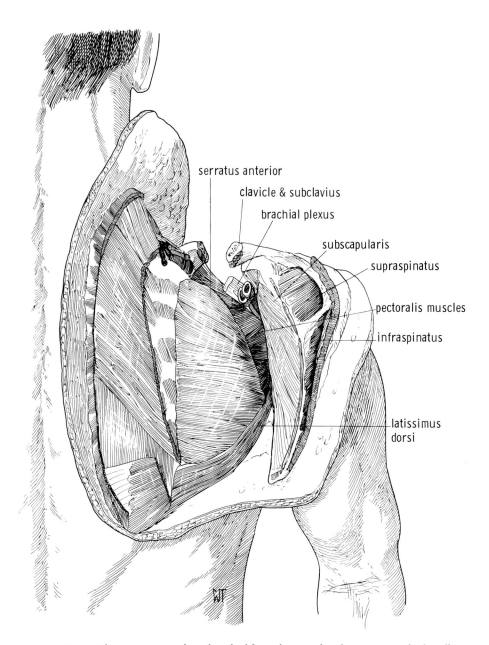

serratus anterior

clavicle & subclavius

brachial plexus

subscapularis

supraspinatus

pectoralis muscles

infraspinatus

latissimus dorsi

Figure 20-5.   The serratus muscle is detached from the scapula. The neurovascular bundle has been divided.

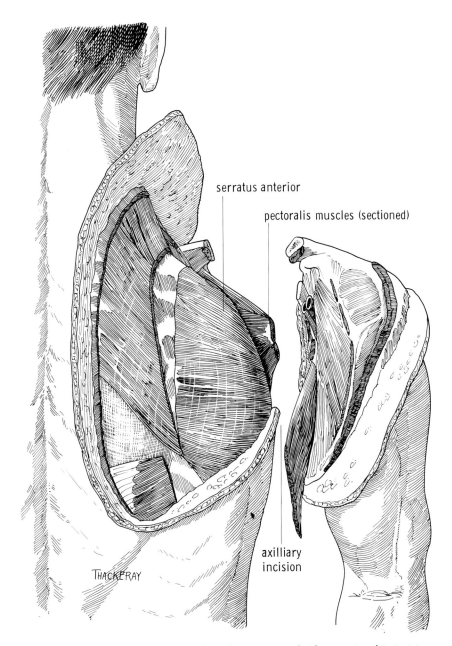

serratus anterior

pectoralis muscles (sectioned)

axilliary
incision

THACKERAY

Figure 20-6. The pectoralis muscles have been sectioned. The anterior skin incision completed, and with it the amputation.

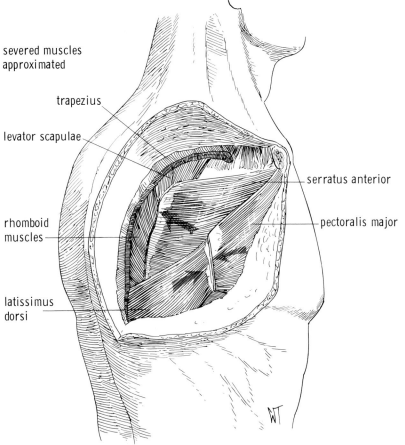

severed muscles
approximated

trapezius

levator scapulae

serratus anterior

pectoralis major

rhomboid
muscles

latissimus
dorsi

Figure 20-7.   The stumps of the muscles have been secured.

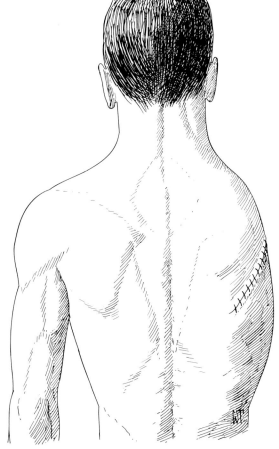

Figure 20-8.   Skin sutures have been completed.

ANTERIOR APPROACH

Technique

After induction of general anesthesia, and with the patient lying on the uninvolved side, the involved upper extremity and adjacent part of the neck and the hemithorax are prepared and draped. The skin incision starts at the junction of the proximal and middle third of the clavicle, and extends along the entire length of the lateral part of the clavicle. The second part of the incision starts at the center of the clavicle, and continues around the anterior axillary fold into the midaxillary line (Fig. 20-9). Through the first part of the incision, the lateral two-thirds of the clavicle are exposed. The lateral part of the clavicular origin of the pectoralis major muscle is released from the clavicle. The central third of the clavicle is exposed subperiostally. It is transected at the lateral border of the insertion of the sternocleidomastoid muscle. By lifting up the clavicle, it is either disarticulated at the acromioclavicular joint or transected further laterally, leaving the acromioclavicular joint intact (Fig. 20-10). Transection of the pectoralis major muscle and release of the pectoralis minor as well as subclavian muscles, bring into view the neu-rovascular bundle (Fig. 20-11). The axillary vein and artery are doubly ligated, clamped, and divided. The omohyoid muscle and brachial plexus are transected next. The suprascapular vein and artery and the transverse cervical artery are ligated and cut (Fig. 20-12).

The skin incision is completed posteriorly by extending it from the acromioclavicular joint slightly medially along the spine of the scapula, and along the medial border of the scapula to its inferior angle (Fig. 20-9). From here, the incision turns laterally and joins the end of the anterior incision at the posterior axillary fold. The trapezius muscle comes into view next, and is transected close to its origin from the spinous processes, exposing the levator scapulae and rhomboid muscles (Fig. 20-13). These are transected as well, allowing anterior movement of the scapula and exposing the serratus anterior muscle and latissimus dorsi (Fig. 20-14), which are transected last (Fig. 20-15). The remaining stumps of the muscles are approximated where possible, or sutured to the soft tissues of the chest wall (Fig. 20-16). Suction drains are inserted into the wound, and the skin flaps are approximated by suturing the subcutaneous tissue with interrupted absorbable sutures, and the skin edges themselves with nonabsorbable sutures (Fig. 20-17).

Figures 20-9 to 20-17.   Fore-quarter amputation, anterior approach.

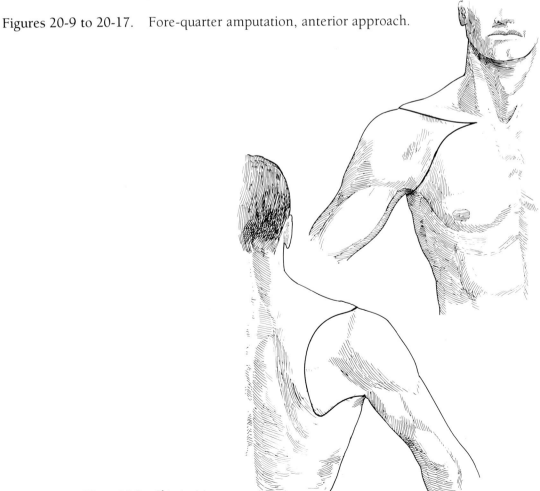

Figure 20-9.   Skin incision.

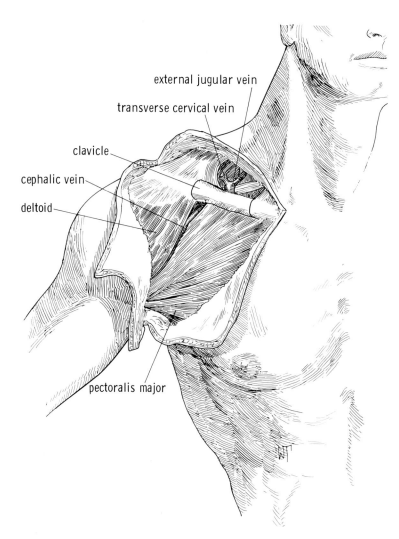

Figure 20-10.   The central portion of the clavicle has been exposed sub-
periostealy and transected.

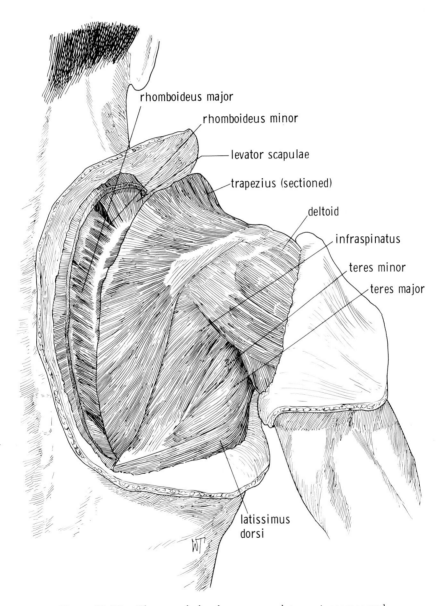

rhomboideus major

rhomboideus minor

levator scapulae

trapezius (sectioned)

deltoid

infraspinatus

teres minor

teres major

latissimus dorsi

Figure 20-13.   The scapula has been exposed, trapezius transected.

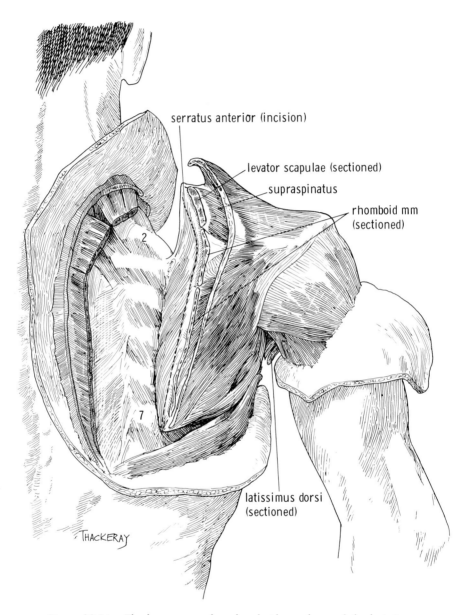

serratus anterior (incision)

levator scapulae (sectioned)

supraspinatus

rhomboid mm
(sectioned)

2

7

latissimus dorsi
(sectioned)

THACKERAY

Figure 20-14.   The levator scapulae, rhomboid muscles, and the latissimus dorsi have been transected. The second and seventh rib are indicated.

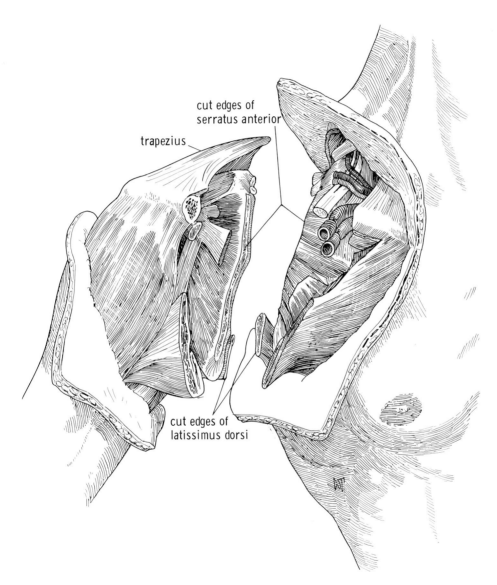

Figure 20-15. After transection of serratus anterior and latissimus dorsi, the amputation is completed.

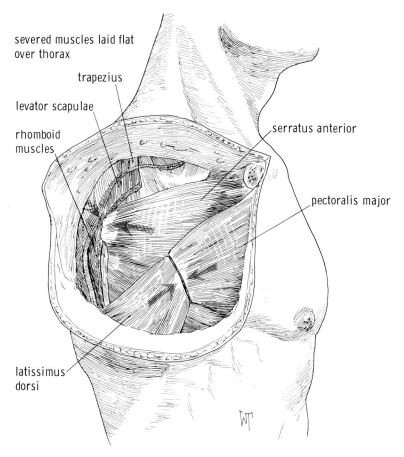

severed muscles laid flat
over thorax

trapezius

levator scapulae

rhomboid
muscles

serratus anterior

pectoralis major

latissimus
dorsi

Figure 20-16.   The stumps of the remaining muscles are attached
to the chest wall.

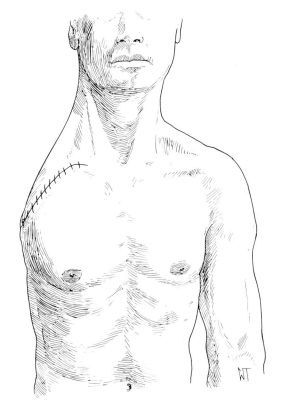

Figure 20-17.   After skin closure, the extreme flattening of the
right shoulder area becomes apparent.

References

1. Pressman PI: Intrascapulothoracic amputation for the complication of breast cancer: A new approach. *Surgery* 75:796–801, 1974.
2. Littlewood H: Amputations at the shoulder and at the hip. *Br Med J* I:381–383, 1922.
3. Pack GT, McNear G, Coley BL: Interscapulothoracic amputation for malignant tumors of the upper extremity. *Surg Gynaecol Obstet* 74:161–175, 1942.
4. Sim FH, Pritchard DJ, Ivins JC: Forequarter amputation. *Orthopaedic Clin North Am* 8(1):921–931, 1977.

Part Three
Postoperative Considerations

CHAPTER 21
Stump Complications

After ablation of a limb, the remaining part is susceptible to a number of problems and complications. In the newly amputated patient, this may lead to a delay in fitting of a prosthesis or may make it impossible to fit one at all. Complications can also make revision or reamputation at a higher level necessary. In the person who already wears a prosthesis, stump diseases may necessitate discontinuation of its use until the disease is cured. This is at best a nuisance and can be, particularly in older people, a disastrous event if the patient cannot get used to renewed wearing of the prosthesis.

The causes for stump diseases can be divided loosely into three groups. However, there is often more than one cause at work. The first group of problems pertains to the stump itself. The most worrisome of these are intrinsic stump problems such as vascular insufficiency, injuries, and particularly fractures and tumors. Another reason for concern is a change in the contour of the stump brought about by a change in the body weight of the patient, by aging, and by stretching of tissues because of inadequate meticulousness in donning the prosthesis.

Stump diseases can also be caused by environmental factors. The dressing on a newly amputated limb might prove too tight and can interfere with the already compromised circulation. In the permanent prosthesis, the altered environment affects mainly the skin. Difficulties in dissipation of heat and moisture in the socket may lead to these changes. The decreased atmospheric pressure in the suction socket can lead to engorgement of the skin and, indeed, the entire distal end of the stump. Other causes are allergic reactions to the materials used in manufacture of the prosthesis.

A third group of causes of stump diseases originates some distance from the original site of amputation. One factor is degenerative disease of joints neighboring the site of amputation. This can lead to an ill-fitting prosthesis because of contractures of those joints or axial deviations. Most of the pain syndromes of the amputation stump are more central in origin, such as nerve root compression in the spine or development of phantom pain.

Therapy for stump disease depends on the diagnosis and, where necessary, identification of the causes. The latter not infrequently requires the cooperation of members of several specialties.

WOUND BREAKDOWN

Under normal circumstances and in the well-vascularized stump, the wound—even of a major amputation—heals surprising well. However, until mature scars have formed between the divided tissues, direct trauma can still lead to a dehiscence of the soft tissue. The healing process is delayed where there is vascular insufficiency. Opening of amputation wounds in these cases can occur even six weeks after surgery. It often occurs after minimal trauma. Another reason for wound breakdown is the presence of a hematoma or an infection with development of an abscess. Neither of them is particularly painful, although abscess formation usually goes along with the general symptoms of infection and sepsis.

Treatment

In the well-vascularized stump, minor wound dehiscences can often be treated by open packing and regular dressing changes until healing by secondary intention has occurred. Where there is a large dehiscence, skin traction may become necessary to counteract retraction of the soft tissues. Where there is gross contamination, the patient may have to undergo additional treatment for formal debridement and packing of the wound. Again, the postoperative treatment of choice is skin traction.

A much greater problem is wound breakdown in a patient with vascular insufficiency. Small areas of wound dehiscence may be caused by local trauma, possibly a small hematoma, and can be treated with dressing changes in the hope for healing by secondary intention. Large areas of wound dehiscence, however, and particularly those that occur many weeks following the amputation, usually indicate insufficient blood supply at the chosen level of amputation; reamputation is often required at a more proximal level.

Large hematomas must be evacuated and the remaining cavity must be treated by open packing. Abscess formation can become a life-threatening situation requiring incision, draining, and open treatment. A common feature of this complication is erosion of the stump of one of the large blood vessels, leading to severe hemorrhage during surgery or, even more dangerously, in the postoperative period.

PROJECTING BONE AND BURSAE

After transection of the bone, there is appositional new bone formation at the cut end of the bony stump. This appositional growth is particularly noticeable in the child amputee, where it can outstrip the growth of the soft tissues surrounding it, leading to erosion of the overlying skin from inside out and, thereby, exposing bony prominences. However, the adult amputee can also develop rather large bony spicules at the stump end. Whereas the child amputee requires stump revision almost regularly — on an average of every two years — new bone formation in the adult hardly ever requires any surgical attention. In the child, stump revision should be done before there is any skin erosion, so that aseptic conditions can be maintained during surgery. The bone is approached through the old incision and is exposed extraperiosteally. The bone is then trimmed back far enough to be covered again by the surrounding soft tissue. Creation of an osteoperiosteal flap to cover the opened marrow cavity or, in the below-knee amputation, to form a bridge between tibia and fibula seems to slow down the appositional growth.

Projecting bone is also an area of concern where disarticulations have been performed. Particularly in the Syme amputation, one can observe the formation of new bone in the heel pad of children as well as adults. This is probably caused by the remaining periosteum of the subperiosteally resected calcaneus. A painful pseudoarthrosis can develop, requiring excision of the ectopic bone.

The development of true bursae with synovial lining leading to discomfort that requires treatment appears to be rare. It has been observed by the author in two cases of amputees with mylodysplasia and below-knee stumps with decreased sensitivity. Both bursae grew to grotesque sizes and had to be resected to allow refitting of prostheses. Inflammation of pre-existing bursae, the olecranon bursa in a Munster socket, and prepatellar and trochanteric bursae in lower extremity amputees can become significant problems, since they require at least modification of the prosthesis. More frequently, however, the solution involves discontinuation of the wearing of the prosthesis until the inflammation of the bursa has receded and no further swelling is present. The bursitis, however, may flare up on subsequent occasions, and excision of the bursa in an inflammation-free interval may become necessary.

INFECTIONS AND ULCERS

In the prosthesis wearer, small infections of the hair follicles do occur. They are usually confined to one or two of the follicles and commonly dry up overnight while the prosthesis is off. More serious is the development of sebaceous cysts in patients with oily skin and heavy hair growth. Sebaceous cysts most often occur at the brim of the prosthesis, where there is more concentrated pressure. These obstructions of the sebaceous glands should be treated carefully with cleaning and expression of the fatty material, since they frequently lead to infections. Where there are several of those cysts, a large abscess can result, leaving the patient without his prosthesis for several weeks, and resulting in a scar in a weight-bearing area, which may require modification of the prosthesis.

The best treatment for both folliculitis and infected sebaceous cysts is prophylaxis. Toughening of the skin of the stump by bathing it in cold water and gently massaging it with loofah sponges may be all that is necessary. If there is a tendency toward sebaceous cysts, baths in hot soapy water may decrease the stagnation in the sebaceous glands. Once a larger abscess forms, discontinuation of wearing of the prosthesis and sometimes limited incision and drainage are necessary.

A common cause for ulcers in the stump is a local or more generalized decrease in the blood supply. The ulcer may develop as a decubitus, and is then found in an area where there is pressure concentration upon the stump within the prosthesis. This pressure can be caused by ridges in the socket itself. It is more often caused by a wrinkle in the stump sock or the socket insert, or by caked powder used too copiously when donning the prosthesis and not removed from the socket. In the patient with known vascular insufficiency, as well as in the aging amputee who lost a limb for other than vascular reasons, the development of ulcerations of the stump should give rise to suspicion of vascular insufficiency. Determination of the pulse volume and measurement of the pressure in the extremity using Doppler give some indication of a circulatory condition of the affected extremity.

The smaller of these ulcerations caused by hypovascularity sometimes heal after prolonged discontinuation of the prosthesis. Changes in the socket alignment and socket insert sometimes prevent reoccurrence of the ulcerations. However, where there are large ulcerations that do not heal readily; stump revision or reamputation at a higher level may ultimately be the treatment of choice.

REDUNDANT SKIN

Following an amputation and after the patient has worn a well-fitting prosthesis for some time, there is a certain amount of atrophy of the subcutaneous soft tissue in the stump. The skin appears less firmly attached to the soft tissue. When the patient dons the prosthesis with little care, the skin is pushed up and will form a roll of skin at the brim of the prosthesis.

The skin roll is particularly bothersome in the patient with an above-knee prosthesis. It is seen at the anteromedial aspect of the upper brim of the prosthesis, and occurs in those patients who gain weight rapidly without changing the size of the socket. Even after weight loss, the skin roll does not readily recede. Procedures for plastic surgery are not desirable, since they leave scars in an area that has to withstand at least some pressure. Thus, a tedious process of providing an extra pocket of room immediately distal to the brim of the prosthesis has to be started. In such cases, a wooden socket is sometimes preferable because of its thicker wall. The patient then has to be taught to meticulously pull the skin roll into the socket to make it reside again within the socket. This process can take many weeks and requires the particular cooperation of the patient.

SKIN DISEASES

A number of skin diseases and skin problems of those parts in and around the socket of the prosthesis can be avoided by meticulous adherence to skin hygiene. The stump inside the socket perspires as much or more than any other part of the body. However, the moisture thus produced does not readily evaporate. The ensuing conditions of moisture, warmth, and darkness are ideal breeding grounds for bacterial and fungal infections.[3,4]

The amputee should therefore make it a regular routine following removal of the prosthesis to wash the stump with soap and water, with the soap prefera-

bly containing a mild bacteriostatic agent. Stump socks should be laundered every day. The socket should be wiped clean at least every other day. After washing the stump, the skin should have enough time to dry and cool down before the prosthesis is donned anew.

Intertrigo

In cases where there are skin folds at the end of the stump either because of pendulous skin or because of irregular scars, a combination of perspiration, constant friction of skin against skin, and accumulation of detritus leads to intertrigo. Similar conditions can occur in the inguinal, perineal, and popliteal region, particularly in the presence of soft tissue rolls. The simplest treatments for this condition are meticulous cleaning in the creases between the soft tissue folds and careful drying. Powders to keep the creases dry may be applied, but their residue has to be removed regularly and carefully.

Dermatitis

Contact dermatitis can occur as the response to an allergic reaction to materials used in the manufacture of the prosthesis. Not only resins and lacquers used to manufacture the socket, but also leather and plastic for external suspensory systems can be the offending agents. The lesions are confined to the area of contact. The therapy, logically, is the removal of the allergenic agent.[1,6] In some cases, this may require extensive changes in components of the prosthesis.

In the patient with eczema, the cause may not be as readily identifiable. If the eczematous lesions of the stump are part of a more generalized eczema, a history of allergy may be elicited. However, all too often this history cannot be obtained. Under those circumstances, local treatment with corticosteroid preparations and drying lotions, if the lesions are weeping, may be the only workable solution.

Epidermoid Inclusion Cysts

Probably because of the persistent friction at the upper end of the prosthesis in the lower limb, minimal trauma occurs at the brim of the lower limb prosthesis. As in microtrauma in the hand, this can lead to implantation of small islands of epithelium into the corium of the skin. Inclusion cysts in the amputee are mainly found in the area around the adductor tendon, the perineum, and the gluteal fold in the above-knee amputee and the anteromedial aspect of the medial tibial plateau in the below-knee amputee. Because of their slow growth, the inclusion cysts become identifiable only many months after the patient has started to wear the prosthesis. They sometimes grow to rather grotesque sizes and become 5 to 6 cm in diameter. Very often, particularly in the thigh, they present only a minor nuisance to a prosthesis wearer. However, not infrequently, the cysts become infected, break open, and drain for long periods of time, preventing the patient from wearing the prosthesis.[2]

There is no satisfactory way of preventing the formation of inclusion cysts. Often, local measures of hot and cold compresses and, where there is an inflammation, local application of corticosteroids upon these cysts may be helpful. Sometimes changes in the alignment of the prosthesis may be sufficient to prevent the formation of new inclusion cysts. All too often, however, incision and drainage of an infected cyst or excision of a large although, not infected, inclusion cyst may become necessary, leaving behind undesirable scars and indurations.

STUMP EDEMA

This problem is almost exclusively confined to the above-knee amputee who is wearing a suction socket. The vacuum created at the end of the prosthesis, and particularly where there is an open chamber, usually exceeds the venous pressure and certainly the pressure in the lymphatic spaces. This leads to an engorgement at the distal end of the stump, with yellowish-brown pigmentation due to capillary breakage. While this condition is almost universal in suction socket wearers, it can lead to further complications that can be prevented. Thus, during the hours out of the prosthesis, the stump end should be dressed in a stump shrinker sock or, less preferably, gently wrapped with an elastic bandage. Attempts should be made to provide some back pressure in the prosthesis by inserting a foam rubber cushion moulded to the contour of the stump end into the bottom of the socket.

If the stump edema continues unchecked, the patient frequently develops a rather leathery, thickened skin at the stump end. This skin frequently acquires cracks and fissures that may become superficially infected. In worse cases, the skin becomes folded on itself, with development of ischemic ulcers that are sometimes of considerable depth. In the patient with stump edema over many years, verrucous hyperplasia can develop. The thickened and grotesquely irregular skin appears to be covered with a multitude of warts. However, even in most of these rather advanced cases, simple compression of the stump end in and out of the prosthesis can lead at least to a decrease and (in some cases) to complete reversal of the condition.[5]

References

1. Correcher BL, Perez AG: Dermatitis from shoes and an amputation prosthesis due to etcaptobenathiazole and paratertiary butyl formaldehyde resin. *Contact Derm* 7:275, 1981.
2. Bendl JB: Painful pigmented prostheses pressure papules. *Cutis* 17:954–957, 1976.
3. DesGroseilliers J-P, Desjardins J-P, Germain J-P, Krol AL: Dermatologic problems in amputees. *CMA J* 118:535–537, 1978.
4. Levy SW: Skin problems of the leg amputee. *Prosthetics and Orthotics Int* 4:37–44, 1980.
5. Levy SW: Disabling skin reactions associated with stump edema. *Int J Dermatol* 16:122–125, 1977.
6. Van Kettel WG: Allergic contact dermatitis of amputation stumps. *Contact Derm* 3:50, 1970.

CHAPTER 22
Pain

PHANTOM LIMB SENSATION

The persistent sensation of the presence of the removed part is to be expected after amputation.[5] The mechanism of the phenomenon is unknown. It apparently requires input from many parts of the nervous system. The sensation itself varies from the feeling of a painless presence of the phantom to extreme pain in it. Although phantom limb sensation appears to be much less pronounced in children, it is nevertheless found, and it can give rise to considerable consternation and fear in the child amputee. There can be no doubt that phantoms are found even in patients with congenital amputations.[9,10]

The phantom limb is frequently felt to be located in a position commensurate with the lost part. The amputee often feels an ability to move the phantom limb voluntarily, and some amputees are able to incorporate the phantom limb into the prosthesis.[1] However, there are amputees who feel their limb distorted and often shortened; particularly after severe accidents and long illnesses preceding the actual amputation, the limb can be felt to be in extreme positions of flexion or extension and immobility.[2,3]

Phantom Limb Pain

The percentage of patients who experience actual pain in the phantom varies considerably among the series examined. Four major properties have been postulated for the phantom limb pain:

1. The pain continues long after actual healing of the amputation wound and can persist for a lifetime.
2. There are trigger zones that, when stimulated, can set off the pain in the phantom limb. The pain can also be triggered by unpleasant experiences or bodily functions.
3. Pain in the phantom limb is more likely to develop in patients who had painful conditions in the affected limb prior to amputation. Phantom limb pain is a continuation of this pain.
4. Mechanical stimulation of the stump, injection of a local anesthetic around a major nerve, or electrical stimulation can, in some cases, relieve the pain for long periods of time.

Attempts at explaining the mechanism that produces pain in a nonexistent part of the body remain speculative. It is unlikely that phantom limb pain is started at a single level of the nervous system, even though surgical procedures involving one single level have occasionally led to lasting success in the suppression of the pain.[6,7,11] Thus, excision of neuromas, conversion of the amputation to a higher level, rhizotomies, and cordotomies, as well as sympathectomies have led to success in some cases. Generally, however, pain recurred after an interval following such procedures.

Any therapy should therefore be more preventative and conservative, rather than surgical. In the patient with long-standing and painful disease in the extremity to be amputated, an effort should be made to produce an extended pain-free interval, possibly through epidural anesthesia. A rigid dressing—even a delayed rigid dressing following amputation—decreases the instance of phantom limb pain. Positive reinforcement and early and vigorous physical therapy following amputation, as well as attempts to involve the patient in the choice and manufacture of the prosthesis, are of value.

In the established case of phantom limb pain, the presence of painful neuromas should be excluded.

Even so, injection of the major nerve trunks is worth trying, since it does seem to relieve the phantom pain in many cases, and sometimes over long periods of time. More important, however, transcutaneous electric nerve stimulation should be tried over a prolonged period of time even though it may not seem successful at the outset.[4]

HYPERAESTHESIA

Almost all amputation stumps have an area of hyperaesthesia extending 1 or 2 cm beyond the amputation scar. Under normal circumstances, this area of hypersensitivity does not interfere with wearing of the prosthesis. There are amputees, however, who complain of large areas of hyperaesthesia in the stump end. These are often caused by transected prefascial skin nerves. Occasionally, however, the hyperaesthesia is caused by circulatory problems either because of vascular disease or because of ill fit and constriction in the socket of the prosthesis.

NEUROMA

Following amputation, all transected nerves develop neuromas. This swelling at the distal end of the transected nerve contains funiculi of nerve fibers in varying orientations that are sharply separated from one another by perineurium. The neuromas can grow to rather grotesque sizes and, on the whole, produce only mild discomfort when subjected to direct pressure or impact. It is therefore inexplicable why some neuromas become extremely painful and even produce symptoms of kausalgia. In some cases, the cause for the discomfort may lie in the fact that the neuroma is caught in the fibrous connective tissue of the scar, thus being subjected to unusual strains. In other cases, neuromas may lie between thin skin coverage and bone, and thus be exposed to undue pressure. In many cases, however, no obvious reason for the pain in the neuroma can be identified.[8]

Numerous methods of treatment of these neuromas have been advocated. Most of them have been found to be unreliable in their efficacy. A number of more helpful methods of treatment have been described in a previous chapter.

References

1. Abramson AS, Feibel A: The phantom phenomenon: Its use and disuse. *Bull NY Acad Med* 57:99–112, 1981.
2. Carlen PL, Wall PD, Nadvorna H, Steinbacht T: Phantom limbs and related phenomena in recent traumatic amputations. *Neurology* 28:211–217, 1978.
3. Henderson WR, Smyth GE: Phantom limbs. *J Neurol Neurosurg Psychol* 11:88–112, 1948.
4. Long DM: Electrical stimulation for the control of pain. *Arch Surg* 112:884–888, 1977.
5. McComas AJ, Sicca REP, Banerjee S: Long term effects of partial limb amputation in man. *J Neurol Neurosurg Psychol* 41:425–432, 1978.
6. Melzack R: Central neural mechanism in pantom limb pain. *Adv Neurol* 4:319–326, 1974.
7. Melzack R, Wall PD: Pain mechanism: A new theory. *Science* 150:971–979, 1965.
8. Omer GE: nerve, neuroma, and pain problems related to upper limb amputations. *Orthopedic Clin North Am* 12:751–762, 1981.
9. Riddoch G: Phantom limbs and body shape. *Brain* 64:197–222, 1941.
10. Weinstein S, Sersen EA, Vetter RJ: Phantoms and somatic sensation in cases of congenital aplasia. *Cortex* 1:276–290, 1967.
11. Weinstein S, Vetter RJ, Sersen EA: The effects of brain damage on the phantom limb. *Cortex* 5:91–103, 1969.

CHAPTER 23
Fractures of the Stump

The factors contributing to fractures of the stump are:

1. Atrophy of the bones and musculature of the amputated limb.
2. An increase in body weight, and thus in the awkwardness of the amputee.
3. In a fall, the lever action of the prosthesis on the body.
4. Lack of mobility in a fall with or without the prosthesis, as well as the absence of an end organ for recovery.

All types of fractures have been observed in the amputated limb. However, spiral fractures are rare in the part of the stump that is covered by the prosthetic socket. This type of fracture is much more common in the part of the limb proximal to the socket. Once the fracture has occurred, the relative loss in muscle power also decreases the amount of displacement that occurs at the fracture site.

Callus formation and consolidation of the fracture are quick. The incidence of pseudoarthrosis is very low, if present at all. On the other hand, malunions are not uncommon and should be avoided, since they lead to faulty weight bearing in the prosthesis.

Since callus formation and consolidation of the fracture are rapid, the therapy should be conservative, if at all possible. Indeed, in many instances, positioning of the fractured limb remnant on a splint is sufficient. Skin traction and skeletal traction are preferable to internal fixation, and impacted femoral neck fractures are best treated with nonweight bearing rather than internal fixation, as long as the position is acceptable for subsequent weight bearing.

Throughout the period of fracture healing, active and vigorous physical therapy is advisable. In particular, the patient with a lower extremity amputation should undergo physical therapy during the period of bedrest in order to maintain strength in the upper extremities in preparation for the time when walking with crutches again becomes possible. Indeed, a rigid-type dressing arrangement may enable the patient to get out of bed early and ambulate with crutches.

In rare instances, open reduction and internal fixation become necessary. It should be kept in mind, however, that the bone and, particularly, the cancellous bone around the joints is atrophic, and that the fixating devices are only able to maintan the alignment. The soft tissue coverage is often poor, and the fixating devices have a tendency to loosen in the bone. Thus, skin traction and skeletal traction are frequently a better way of maintaining the alignment of the fracture until the callus formation is sufficient to maintain the alignment without external support.

References

1. Freese P: Frakturen an Amputationsstümpfen und amputierten Gliedmassen. *Monatsschrift für Unfallheilkunde* 68:433–439, 1975.
2. Lewallen RP, Johnson EW: Fractures in amputation stumps. *Mayo Clin Proc* 56:22–26, 1981.
3. Napieralski K: Frakturen an amputierten Extremitäten. *Zentralblatt für Chirurgie* 91:302–308, 1966.

CHAPTER 24
Reamputation and Revision

The technique of reamputation—conversion of an amputation to a higher level—generally follows the principles of any amputation at that particular level. In the patient with a Syme amputation, conversion to a below-knee level would follow the principles of below-knee amputation, and so forth. However, for the patient, such a procedure represents another extensive procedure and demands the necessary physical resilience. In addition, reamputation again places psychological burden upon the patient; having gone through readjustment to the loss of a limb, the patient once again must face the same demand. Added to this is the almost inherent worry that since one amputation has not worked to eliminate the disease, the second one may not work either—and that this is only the second step in a downhill course.

Even more than the patient undergoing primary amputation, the patient slated for reamputation will need psychological support and understanding to oversome this predicament. If possible, the patient should be given a plan of postoperative treatment so that a sense of predictability is restored.

INDICATIONS FOR REVISONS

Amputations are revised either to rearrange soft tissue, or to remove additional parts of the bone. Rearrangement of soft tissue coverage at the end of the stump is usually done for patients with adherent and irregular scars, or in cases where a circular open amputation has been performed. The procedure begins with the excision of the scar, saving as much viable skin as possible. The underlying, usually rather extensive, fibrous tissue has to be excised down to the bone. Where possible, the musculature should be mobilized and brought down to provide adequate soft tissue coverage. To this end, the scar tissue has to be removed back to bleeding tissue. The skin overlying the muscle has to be elevated with a sufficiently thick layer of subcutaneous tissue over a distance of 3 to 4 cm. Skin closure should be possible under a minimal amount of tension.

Revisions where in addition to removal and rearrangement of the soft tissue the bone has to be removed commonly become necessary in children when diaphyseal overgrowth threatens to perforate the skin at the end of the stump. In these cases, the scar at the end of the stump is excised. The end of the bone is exposed extraperiosteally and resected, leaving an osteoperiosteal flap to cover the marrow cavity. Since some of the bulk of the bone has been removed, the approximation of soft tissue and skin closure is usually a simple matter.

Index